The Ghost in the Cancer

Towards a New Science of Radiation Oncology

R. Vaitheeswaran, PhD

notionpress.com

INDIA • SINGAPORE • MALAYSIA

ISBN
Paperback 979-8-90362-916-9
Hardrcase 979-8-90479-594-8

E- mail id: vaithe1985@gmail.com

*For my parents, **R. Bhanumathi** and **V. Ranganathan**,*
with deepest love and gratitude

Contents

Preface

Radiotherapy is one of medicine's great triumphs of precision. We learned to see tumors with extraordinary clarity. We learned to sculpt radiation beams around them with millimetric accuracy, threading dose through healthy tissue to reach a target with a faithfulness that would have seemed impossible a generation ago. And with each step forward in that precision, outcomes improved.

Then consider this.

Two patients. Same cancer. Same stage. Same carefully optimized treatment plan. One responds. The other does not.

This is not a rare event. It is not a statistical curiosity confined to the tails of a distribution. It is a recurring feature of clinical reality, familiar to every radiation oncologist who has practiced long enough to follow their patients through years of treatment and aftermath. The plan was right. The delivery was accurate. And yet the system did not behave as expected.

The conventional answer to this puzzle is biological variability—the natural spread in how tumors respond, the stochastic noise of cells and molecules. This answer is not wrong. But it is incomplete. Because variability of this kind, if it were purely random, should average out. It should not produce the systematic, patterned anomalies that radiobiology has struggled to explain for decades.

Something else is going on.

This book argues that what is going on has a precise name, even if it does not yet appear in textbooks. Beneath the images we acquire, the dose distributions we calculate, and the response curves we measure, there is a deeper structure—a hidden state that shapes how a tumor evolves and responds, but that is never directly seen. It is not mysterious. It is not supernatural. It is simply unmeasured. And because it is unmeasured, our models—however sophisticated—are models of a projection, not of the thing itself.

We will call this hidden structure the ghost in the cancer.

The name is a metaphor, but the concept is not. Hidden states are a well-established feature of complex dynamical systems. In control engineering, in neuroscience, in economics, the recognition that a system's observable outputs do not uniquely determine its internal configuration is not a philosophical speculation—it is a mathematical fact (Bellman and Åström, 1970; Villaverde et al., 2016). You can observe everything that is measurable and still not know the state of the system. The ghost is the part of the state space you cannot see. It is like evaluating a chess position with half the board hidden—what is visible is correct, but not sufficient to determine what the position is.

In tumors, this hidden state evolves over time. It integrates the history of prior exposures. It constrains which future behaviors the system can adopt. And it means that the same treatment, applied under apparently identical conditions, need not produce the same outcome—not because the system is random, but because it is not fully observed.

Once you take this idea seriously, several of radiotherapy's most persistent puzzles begin to look different. Why does delivering the same dose at an ultra-high rate spare normal tissue in ways that conventional delivery cannot? Why does redistributing dose across space—leaving large regions deliberately untreated—sometimes produce better tumor control than uniform irradiation? Why does increasing dose per fraction, beyond a certain threshold, generate effects that no current model reliably predicts?

These are typically treated as three separate problems, each requiring its own biological explanation. This book argues they are not separate at all. They are signals—signals of the same underlying reality, visible along three different axes of intervention. Together, they reveal that the tumor is not the static target that conventional radiobiology imagines. It is a dynamical system with memory, governed by a hidden state, partially observable at best.

That recognition changes the problem entirely. If we are right, then the central question of radiotherapy is not simply what dose to deliver. It is what state the system is in—and how we can guide it. The two questions look similar on the surface. Beneath the surface, they require completely different frameworks, different tools, and a different philosophy of what it means to treat a cancer.

This book builds that framework. It draws on radiobiology, systems biology, information theory, the neuroscience of inference under uncertainty, evolutionary game theory, and the emerging science of biological memory and cognition. The mathematics that underpins the full theory is developed in Appendix A, for those who want it. The main text is written for readers who want the argument—clinicians and physicists alike—without needing to follow every derivation.

What makes this book possible now, in a way it would not have been five years ago, is that the key theoretical claim—that biological networks learn their environment and encode that learning as organisational state—has moved from inference to experiment. Pigozzi et al. (2025) showed that gene regulatory networks learn associations in the precise Pavlovian sense, and that learning measurably reorganises the network into a more integrated whole. Doan et al. (2026) showed the same in a single cell with no nervous system whatsoever. The tumour's capacity to learn its treatment is no longer a theoretical claim. It is a demonstrated biological fact. This book is the first to ask what that fact implies for how we treat cancer with radiation.

The ghost, it turns out, can be tracked. It leaves traces in the patterns of response that our current models cannot explain. And if it can be tracked, it can—in principle—be influenced. Not by delivering more dose, but by understanding the system more deeply, and acting on that understanding with a new kind of intelligence. That is where this book ends. But it begins here, with the simplest and most stubborn fact in all of radiotherapy: that two patients, treated identically, can follow entirely different paths.

The difference is the ghost. And it is time to stop ignoring it.

Acknowledgements

Every book has a origin story. This one begins with a girl I never spoke to.

It was the day of admissions to the MSc Medical Physics programme. I had already made up my mind: Material Science. It seemed the sensible choice—respectable, employable, comprehensible to relatives. I was standing at the notice board, pen in hand, about to commit, when I noticed a young woman nearby reading the same list. She was weeping. Not discreetly. Genuinely weeping—the kind that suggests the world has just arranged itself against you in a particularly personal way. She had not made the cut for Medical Physics.

Something shifted in me at that moment. I am not sure whether it was empathy, curiosity, or simply the mild superstition that anything capable of producing that much feeling must be worth investigating. I put down Material Science and chose Medical Physics instead.

I never learned her name. I never saw her again. But she is, in a very real sense, the reason this book exists. Wherever she is, I hope her own path led somewhere equally unexpected.

The second turn came during my MSc project, and I will confess it was powered less by intellectual ambition than by a strong reluctance to travel. The project required fieldwork in Delhi. Delhi is far from Attur—a small town in Salem district, Tamil Nadu, which is where I come from, and which is exactly as far from Delhi as it sounds. The journey would have been long. The summer would have been hot. The logistics would have been considerable.

I went to my project supervisor, Dr. Aruna, and made what I privately considered a compelling case: I would stay back and do a theoretical project instead. This was, it should be noted, approximately twenty years before theoretical work in medical physics MSc projects was anything approaching normal. Dr. Aruna listened to my argument with the gracious patience of someone who has seen many students attempt creative interpretations of academic requirements. She agreed—though not, I suspect, without some private reservations about what exactly I would produce.

She was right to be sceptical, at least initially. The project ran into a mathematical wall almost immediately—an integral that I could not crack and that the entire theoretical structure depended on. In desperation, I turned to my cousin Siva, who has the kind of relationship with mathematics that most people reserve for breathing: effortless, continuous, and slightly alarming to witness. He looked at the integral, solved it in what seemed like an indecently short time, and handed it back. That integral was the hinge on which the project turned. Siva has no formal connection to medical physics. He simply happened to be a genius in the right place at the right time, and I owe him more than he probably realises.

To Dr. Aruna, who gave a lazy student a chance he did not entirely deserve and made him work harder than he expected: thank you.

In the field, I had the extraordinary good fortune of finding a guru in the truest sense of the word. Dr. Sathiya Narayanan is one of the most respected and widely known medical physicists in this country, and he shaped the way I think about the discipline at every level—not just technically, but in terms of what the practice is actually for, what it demands of the people who do it, and what it means to do it well. Everything I know that is worth knowing in medical physics passes through what I learned from him.

My PhD supervisor, Dr. Maria Das, another well-known figure in the medical physics community in the country, gave me something different but equally essential: systematic rigour. Research without structure is speculation. Dr. Das taught me the difference, and did so with the kind of patient, precise guidance that turns a student who thinks he understands something into a researcher who actually does. I owe these two mentors everything that is careful and disciplined in this book. What remains careless is entirely my own contribution.

I also owe a particular debt to Dr. Kumaraswamy—one of the most prominent radiation oncologists in India—for a shared failure that, fifteen years later, I have come to regard as one of the most instructive experiences of my career.

It was early in my time in the field. Dr. Kumaraswamy and I had a hypothesis: that the Hounsfield Unit values obtained from CT imaging might carry information about tumour response to treatment—that something in the way the CT numbers shifted over the course of radiotherapy might tell us something about how the biology was changing. It was, looking back, an early and intuitive attempt to find the hidden signal that this book is about.

We tried. We had a head and neck case, approximately thirty serial CT scans acquired using what was then a cutting-edge CT-on-rails system, and two researchers who were convinced they were on the verge of something. We were not. Nothing useful came from it. The data refused to yield what we were looking for, and eventually we accepted that the signal—if it existed—was not in the Hounsfield numbers at all, or at least not accessible to us with that technology.

Fifteen years later, I find myself writing about MR-Linacs and apparent diffusion coefficient mapping and the possibility of using serial diffusion-weighted imaging to track organisational state changes in real time during treatment. ADC—the signal in diffusion-weighted MRI—is almost certainly what we were actually looking for back then, in that head and neck case, with those thirty CT scans and our misplaced confidence in Hounsfield Units.

We were asking the right question. We simply had the wrong instrument. I am grateful to Dr. Kumaraswamy for asking it with me, and for being the kind of clinician who thinks it is worth asking at all.

The ideas in this book were also shaped by conversations, challenges, and encounters too numerous to fully catalogue—with colleagues, students, and patients whose questions taught me more than I often recognised at the time. To all of them: thank you.

The book was written across several years that included, among other things, a pandemic, a period of personal difficulty, and the slower, ongoing effort to find a framework adequate to a problem I had been circling for a long time. That it exists at all is due in part to the patience of everyone who waited while I worked, and in part to the conviction—sometimes stronger, sometimes weaker—that the ghost in the cancer was real, and worth pursuing.

A Note Before You Begin

This book started in 2019 with a theory of consciousness.

Not because I was working on consciousness. I am a medical physicist—my world is radiation, dose, treatment planning, etc. But I read about Integrated Information Theory, and something in it refused to leave me alone. The idea that a system's causal structure—not its components, not its chemistry, but the way its parts constrain each other—could be the primary object of a science. I didn't know what to do with that. I just knew it felt important.

Then I read Paul Davies. And somewhere in the argument about information as a causal force in biology, something clicked. Not loudly. More like a door opening onto a room I hadn't known was there. Davies introduced the concept of target morphology—the idea that biological tissue carries a representation of the organisational form it is trying to maintain or recover. I read it as a developmental biology concept, and filed it away with a vague intuition that it might apply more broadly—to tissue under stress, perhaps, or to tissue under treatment. I didn't know yet how to make that precise. I just kept pulling the thread.

I was not aware, when I began, that radiobiology was failing in FLASH, in spatially fractionated radiotherapy, or in stereotactic body radiotherapy. Those anomalies came later. What I had in 2019 was only an idea about organisational state and a suspicion that it might matter for how tumors respond to radiation. The framework sat incomplete for years—waiting, as it turned out, for evidence that did not yet exist.

Then 2021 arrived.

My mother and I both contracted COVID-19. I will not dwell on what that year was. What I will say is that when I came back to this work—and it took months before I could even try—I could not find it. Not the files, not the argument, not the thread I had been following. I spent the better part of a year simply reconstructing what I had done. Reading my own notes as though someone else had written them. Trying to remember why I had believed any of this mattered.

In 2023, my mother suffered a heart attack. I will not pretend that left the work unaffected. There are losses that don't just take time—they take the quieter conviction that any of it matters. I found my way back slowly. The work waited.

I still did not have the mathematical architecture the framework required. The Free Energy Principle entered late, and without it the control framework of Part IV could not be built. And the biological evidence for non-neural learning—which would become the empirical foundation for the book's central claim—did not yet exist.

It arrived in 2025.

When I read the papers on associative conditioning in gene regulatory networks and single-cell memory, I was not looking for confirmation of a theory. I was asking a narrower question: could this biology explain the FLASH effect? The answer led somewhere I had not anticipated. FLASH, spatially fractionated radiotherapy, stereotactic body radiotherapy—three clinical anomalies I had been aware of separately—suddenly resolved into a single picture. The same hidden structure, visible from three different angles. That convergence was not something I planned or predicted. It revealed itself. I am still not entirely sure I deserved to find it.

And then, following that thread, I found Michael Levin's experimental work.

I had encountered the concept of target morphology in Davies years earlier and had sensed, without being able to make it precise, that it might apply to tissue organisation more broadly. What I had not known was that Levin had already spent years demonstrating exactly this—experimentally, in living tissue—showing that bioelectric fields encode organisational memory, that this memory governs cellular behaviour by overriding genetic programming, and that it can be deliberately altered through physiological means without touching the genome. He had proven, in planaria and in cancer models, what I had only been able to theorise. The connection between what I had proposed and what he had shown was not something I had planned for. It was the most surprising moment in six years of work—the discovery that the ghost had already been found, by someone who hadn't been looking for it in radiotherapy at all.

I am telling you all of this not for sympathy but for honesty. Because the book you are about to read makes arguments with a confidence that the process of writing it did not always possess. There were long stretches when the framework was incomplete, when the evidence was missing, when I was simply lost. The doubt was not occasional—it was the default condition. What kept me going was not confidence in my own ability to finish this, but the conviction that the problem itself was real. That the ghost in the cancer is not a metaphor. That tumors are being treated as static targets when they are dynamical systems with memory, and that this mismatch is costing lives in ways that more dose and better imaging will not fix.

Whether this specific framework is the right response to that problem is for science to determine. The predictions are registered in Appendix D. I have tried to be honest throughout about what is established and what remains a disciplined what-if.

But the problem is real. Of that I have not had a single moment of doubt.

This book is the result of six years of work—interrupted, resumed, partially lost, rebuilt—by one medical physicist who started with a theory of consciousness and ended up here. It is offered in that spirit: not as a finished answer, but as a serious attempt to ask the right question.

R. Vaitheeswaran 2026

E- mail id: vaithe1985@gmail.com

A Brief History of Radiotherapy

The story of how radiotherapy became what it is today begins not with a plan but with an accident.

On the 8th of November 1895, Wilhelm Röntgen noticed that a fluorescent screen across his darkened laboratory was glowing even though it lay outside the path of his cathode ray tube. The tube was enclosed. The screen had no business glowing. He spent the next seven weeks in near isolation, barely leaving the laboratory, trying to understand what he had found. He called it X-radiation—X for unknown. Within weeks, physicians across Europe were imaging bones. Within two months, the first cancer patient had been treated with X-rays—not by a physician but by a medical student in Chicago named Emile Grubbé, who had been manufacturing X-ray tubes as a small business and noticed that his own hands were becoming inflamed (Orton, 2022). The gap between the discovery of a new physical phenomenon and its clinical application was measured in weeks. Radiotherapy was born not from systematic science but from urgency and opportunism—a pattern that would recur throughout its history.

The Fractionation Wars

For the first two decades of radiotherapy, the field was divided by a dispute that sounds almost comic in retrospect but was fiercely contested at the time.

The Erlangen School, led by Hermann Wintz in Germany, held that single large doses were the correct approach. Fractionated treatment—dividing the total dose into multiple smaller sessions over days or weeks—was, in Wintz's words, "weak" and "primitive." The Paris School, led by Henri Coutard at the Radium Institute, held the opposite view and had been practising fractionated radiotherapy since 1919 (Thames, 1988). The argument continued, increasingly acrimonious, across the 1920s.

Then Claudius Regaud—a researcher who had been studying spermatogenesis in rams—ran the experiment that settled the matter. He found that he could sterilise a ram's testes with fractionated radiation delivered in three sessions fifteen days apart, while leaving the scrotal skin intact. With a single large dose, he could not achieve both. The skin would be destroyed before the testes were sterilised (Regaud, 1922). The implication was immediate: fractionation was not weakness. It was the mechanism by which the therapeutic window between tumour and normal tissue could be opened. By 1932, when Coutard published his results treating head and neck cancers with protracted fractionated radiotherapy, the single-dose school had effectively conceded (Coutard, 1932). The field had its organising principle—derived from a ram, formalised in a Paris basement, and clinical practice was changed forever.

A War Changes Everything

World War II interrupted radiotherapy practice across Europe. But it did something else that none of its participants anticipated: it created the conditions for a fundamental transformation in the biological understanding of radiation.

The atomic bombings of Hiroshima and Nagasaki in August 1945 produced, among their catastrophic human consequences, the largest involuntary radiation biology experiment in history. Within six weeks, research teams were in both cities documenting biological effects. In November 1946, President Truman approved the creation of the Atomic Bomb Casualty Commission—later the Radiation Effects Research Foundation—which would follow approximately 120,000 survivors for decades (RERF, 2007). The data that emerged established dose-response relationships for leukaemia, solid tumours, and a range of other effects that became the empirical foundation of modern radiation biology and protection (Grant et al., 2012).

The war also accelerated the technology. The Manhattan Project's investment in particle physics produced accelerators, expertise in high-energy beams, and an entire generation of physicists who redirected their knowledge toward medicine. The first hospital-based linear accelerator for patient treatment was installed at Stanford in 1956 (Bernier et al., 2004).

There was a further irony that nobody planned for. The wartime research into radiation damage—driven by the urgent need to understand what atomic weapons did to human tissue—generated the cellular and molecular biology that gave radiotherapy its theoretical foundation. The four Rs of radiobiology—repair, repopulation, redistribution, reoxygenation—emerged from laboratory work whose urgency was inseparable from the post-war political moment (Withers, 1975). Science rarely develops in straight lines. The history of radiotherapy is in large part a history of knowledge borrowed from contexts that had nothing to do with cancer.

Building the Model: A Wartime Equation Becomes Clinical Currency

The linear-quadratic model—the mathematical framework that still governs clinical radiobiology—has its own wartime origin. Douglas Lea and his colleague D.G. Catcheside, working in Cambridge during the early 1940s, fitted chromosome aberration data to an expression of the form $\alpha D + \beta D^2$—where α and β captured two distinct mechanisms of radiation-induced cell killing (Lea and Catcheside, 1942). Their paper, published in the Journal of Genetics in 1942, was concerned with fundamental radiobiology, not clinical practice. That it would eventually become the central tool of clinical dose calculation was something neither author could have anticipated.

The model was initially neglected. It took decades of subsequent work—by Kellerer and Rossi (1972) refining the biophysical theory, by Chadwick and Leenhouts (1973) deriving it from molecular damage mechanisms, and ultimately by Jack Fowler, whose 1989 synthesis in the British Journal of Radiology made the biologically effective dose the common currency of clinical radiobiology—before Lea and Catcheside's wartime observation became the framework that every radiation oncologist now uses to compare fractionation schedules (Fowler, 1989).

The model's elegance is genuine. Within its domain—conventional fractionation, modest doses per fraction, standard dose rates—it provides a reliable and clinically validated approximation that has served the field for decades. Its limits become apparent only when the conditions that defined its derivation are systematically exceeded. That is a story the chapters ahead will tell in full.

The Technical Revolution: When Other Industries Came to the Clinic

By the 1970s and 1980s, the dominant challenge in radiotherapy had shifted from biology to geometry. Computed tomography—developed by Hounsfield and Cormack, who shared the Nobel Prize in Physiology or Medicine in 1979—gave radiation oncologists three-dimensional visualisation of tumours for the first time. Treatment planning could now account for the actual shape of the target and the anatomy of the organs surrounding it. The multileaf collimator, refined through the 1980s, allowed the radiation beam to be shaped dynamically during delivery, conforming dose to complex target volumes with millimetre precision.

The next generation of image verification came from an unexpected direction entirely. The electronic portal imaging devices that began replacing film-based verification in the late 1980s used flat-panel detector technology built around amorphous silicon thin-film transistor arrays—the same TFT-on-glass fabrication process that underpins every laptop screen and LCD monitor (Antonuk et al., 1992). The clinical radiotherapy community did not develop this technology. It inherited it from the consumer electronics industry, whose investment in display manufacturing had—largely inadvertently—created the component that would allow real-time patient positioning verification during treatment (Antonuk, 2002). The flat-panel EPID mounted on the treatment gantry and the screen of the clinician's laptop share the same fundamental fabrication lineage.

This pattern—technology developed for one purpose finding transformative application in radiotherapy—runs throughout the field's history. Accelerator physics developed for nuclear research gave hospitals their linear accelerators. Semiconductor manufacturing developed for consumer displays gave clinics their digital imaging. Magnetic resonance technology developed for chemistry and neuroscience gave radiotherapy its soft-tissue visualisation. The MR-linac—integrating real-time MRI with radiation delivery—is the most recent expression of this borrowing, and it is the platform on which the measurement instruments proposed in this book would operate.

The Accumulation of Precision—and Its Limits

By the early twenty-first century, radiotherapy had built an extraordinary technical edifice. More precise machines. More detailed biological models. More sophisticated planning algorithms. More accurate delivery. And at each step, outcomes improved.

But the improvements were not proportional to the investment, and certain failures proved stubbornly resistant to technical solutions. Escalating dose did not eliminate recurrence at the rates the models predicted. More accurate delivery did not fully close the gap between patients who responded and patients who did not. The biology was doing something the framework was not representing.

Three specific domains crystallised this gap in ways that pointed not toward better engineering but toward a different kind of understanding. They are the subject of the chapters that follow—and the convergence between them is what this book is about.

PART I

The Problem We Cannot Fully Explain

CHAPTER

01

The Problem the Model Cannot See

Radiotherapy is one of medicine's most precise instruments. We can image a tumour to the millimetre, sculpt a dose distribution around it with sub-millimetre accuracy, and deliver that distribution to within a few percent of what we planned. The physics is correct. The geometry is correct. The plan is correct.

And yet the cancer comes back.

Not rarely. Not in exceptional cases. Local recurrence after radiotherapy—in lung, in head and neck, in cervix, in rectum, in prostate—occurs at rates that have proven stubbornly resistant to improvement despite decades of technical refinement (Joiner and van der Kogel, 2018). The delivery became more accurate. The imaging became more detailed. The planning algorithms became more sophisticated. And recurrence persisted, in forms that the framework used to design the treatment could not predict.

This book is about why. Not in general—about why in radiotherapy specifically, and about what the failure of prediction reveals about what is missing from the radiobiological framework we use.

The Two-Patient Problem

Begin with the observation every radiation oncologist knows. Two patients. Same cancer. Same stage. Same histology. Same carefully optimised treatment plan, delivered with equivalent accuracy to both. One responds. The tumour shrinks, disappears on imaging, and does not return. The other responds initially—the scan at the midpoint of treatment looks encouraging—and then, months or years later, disease returns. Not at a distant site. At the treated site. The tumour that appeared to respond did not respond lastingly. Something survived that should not have survived. Something adapted that the treatment should not have allowed to adapt.

The conventional radiobiological explanation is straightforward: a resistant subpopulation of cells survived the treatment. Cells with reduced oxygenation, enhanced DNA repair capacity, or intrinsically lower radiosensitivity were present from the outset and persisted through what killed the rest (Hall and Giaccia, 2012). Recurrence, on this account, is incomplete eradication—a counting problem, solved in principle by delivering more dose, more accurately, to a better-defined target.

This explanation is not wrong. But it is incomplete in a way that matters enormously. If recurrence were primarily a problem of surviving resistant clones, then progressively improving dose delivery, targeting accuracy, and tumour coverage should progressively reduce it. It has not done so at the rates the model predicts (Joiner and van der Kogel, 2018). And the variability—the fact that two patients with apparently identical tumours follow entirely different trajectories—persists across tumour types, treatment centres, and generations of technical improvement in ways that dose escalation and targeting precision alone do not fully account for (Fowler, 2010).

This persistence of unexplained variability suggests that something else is determining which patient responds and which does not—something the treatment plan does not account for and the model does not represent.

Resistance Is Not Static

The deeper difficulty is what recurrence reveals about the nature of resistance. Tumours that return after radiotherapy do not simply reassert the biology they had before treatment. They return differently—with altered sensitivity profiles, changed growth patterns, and responses to subsequent treatment that cannot be predicted from initial characteristics (Greaves and Maley, 2012). This is not the behaviour of a pre-existing subpopulation that was always going to survive. It is the behaviour of a system that has changed.

Radiation selects for cells with reduced oxygenation and lower intrinsic radiosensitivity (Gray et al., 1953). It activates pro-survival signalling pathways (Hanahan and Weinberg, 2011) and upregulates DNA damage repair in surviving cells (Jeggo and Löbrich, 2007). These mechanisms are real and well-documented. But look past the individual mechanisms and a pattern emerges that they do not individually explain.

Resistance is directional. It does not drift randomly. It moves, consistently and reliably, toward configurations that are better adapted to the specific treatment being applied—calibrated to the dose levels, fractionation patterns, and delivery characteristics of the treatment actually used (Gatenby and Gillies, 2009; Greaves and Maley, 2012). When the treatment changes, resistance frequently follows—adapting to the new pressure with a specificity that is difficult to explain if adaptation is purely stochastic. A fixed, predictable treatment policy is, in effect, a learnable signal. Not in the sense of intention or awareness, but in the same way any adaptive system changes when exposed to a repeated pattern—what is applied consistently becomes what the system is shaped to handle. And there is growing evidence that biological systems under persistent selective pressure do something that resembles learning it (Gatenby et al., 2009; Zhang et al., 2017).

Anyone who has spent time around a small child will recognise the pattern. My niece Vedha, at four, when told she can have only one chocolate, does not simply accept the limit. She asks me, gets a no, and immediately asks her mother as though it has not been settled. When that fails, she returns later, points to the wrapper, and asks again for "one chocolate." If refused, she waits, tries again in a different tone—and when all else fails, escalates to tears. We know it is a performance. It works often enough to be worth trying. Within a few iterations, she has not just encountered the rule—she has learned how it is enforced, and she reliably ends up with more than one.

Over time, we learned this pattern and do something different. When she starts asking again, we do not repeat the rule. We change the interaction—a story, a distraction, a shift in attention. The request is not negotiated; it is dissolved. What stops the behaviour is not a stronger rule, but a change in what the system is engaging with.

Radiotherapy faces the same problem. A fixed, repeatable treatment policy is not just applied to the tumour; it is learned by it. If the system is adapting to the structure of what we deliver, then control requires changing that structure—not simply increasing the dose, but altering the way the system is engaged.

The clinical implication is uncomfortable but important. The harder and more predictably you push with a fixed strategy, the faster the tumour's adaptive dynamics can process the information in that strategy and reorganise accordingly. Maximum tolerated dose, delivered continuously in a fixed pattern until progression, may be the most informative signal you can give a system that is learning to evade it.

We will return to this at length in Part IV. For now, one observation is sufficient: the directionality of resistance, and its calibration to the specific treatment applied, suggests that something within the tumour is integrating the information content of the treatment signal—not consciously, not intentionally, but in the same functional sense that any adaptive system processes information from its environment. The framework we use to plan and deliver radiotherapy has no representation of this process. It models dose and damage. It does not model what the tumour does with what it learns.

What the Radiobiological Model Can and Cannot See

The linear-quadratic model—the mathematical framework that governs clinical radiobiology—has served the field for decades and serves it still. Within its domain of validity: modest doses per fraction, conventional delivery rates, spatially uniform irradiation across a well-characterised target, it provides a reliable and clinically validated approximation (Fowler, 1989). The model captures the essential radiobiology of repair, repopulation, redistribution, and reoxygenation—the four Rs that have organised clinical fractionation since the post-war era (Withers, 1975). Its clinical utility is genuine and not in dispute here.

What is in dispute is its completeness—specifically, whether the model's mathematical structure is capable of representing all the biologically relevant features of tumour response to radiation. And the answer that is about to unfold in the coming chapters, as three specific experimental and clinical phenomena have made increasingly clear, is no.

The model treats dose as the primary determinant of biological response. It treats each fraction as an independent event. It treats each spatial region of the tumour as responding to its own local dose without reference to what is happening elsewhere. And it treats radiosensitivity parameters—alpha and beta—as fixed tissue constants rather than as quantities that might depend on the tumour's internal condition at the time of irradiation.

Each of these views is an assumption. And each assumption, it turns out, fails under conditions that modern radiotherapy has begun to explore—conditions that push the three fundamental dimensions of radiation delivery to their extremes.

Three Windows

Radiation can be varied along three and only three fundamental axes: when it is delivered, where it is delivered, and how much is delivered. Time, space, and magnitude.

In recent years, three clinical and experimental phenomena have independently cracked the radiobiological model open—one along each axis.

When radiation is delivered at ultra-high dose rates—completing a therapeutic dose in a fraction of a second rather than several minutes—normal tissue is spared in ways that the LQ model does not predict and cannot reproduce (Favaudon et al., 2014; Vozenin et al., 2019). The phenomenon is called FLASH. It is not an artifact. It has been confirmed across multiple species, multiple tissue types, and multiple irradiation modalities. And what it reveals is that the rate and temporal structure of delivery—variables the LQ model treats as biologically irrelevant—change the biological outcome in ways that depend on something the model has no representation of.

When radiation is delivered in a spatially non-uniform pattern—high-dose peaks alternating with low-dose or zero-dose valleys across the tumour volume—tumour regions that received little or no dose respond as though they had been treated (Mohiuddin et al., 1999; Griffin et al., 2020). The phenomenon is called spatially fractionated radiotherapy, or SFRT. It violates the assumption that tumour regions respond only to their own local dose. It reveals that the tumour is a coupled spatial system—that perturbations propagate between regions in ways that the LQ model's assumption of spatial independence cannot accommodate.

When radiation is delivered at very high doses per fraction—the regime of stereotactic body radiotherapy—the model's predictions become unreliable in ways that cannot be corrected by adjusting its parameters (Fowler, 2010; Kirkpatrick et al., 2008; Astrahan, 2008). The survival curve straightens beyond a transition dose. BED calculations become unstable. Outcome variability across patients persists and exceeds what the model attributes to known sources of biological spread. The model breaks down not gradually but qualitatively—a regime transition, not a scaling error.

Three axes. Three failures. Each failure is a place where the model's assumptions give out under pressure.

One Pattern—and One Hidden Cause

These three phenomena are typically studied by separate research communities, discussed in separate literatures, and treated as separate technical problems. FLASH has its oxygen depletion hypotheses. SFRT has its bystander effect and immune activation literature. SBRT has its LQ-linear extensions and universal survival curve alternatives.

This book argues that framing is wrong. The three phenomena are not separate problems. They are three projections of the same underlying reality—three places where the same structural limitation of the model becomes undeniable, each visible along a different axis of intervention.

What they share is this: in each case, biological response depends on context that the LQ model has no variable to represent. The model maps inputs to outputs through fixed relationships. It has no internal configuration—no state—that evolves over time and shapes how each new input is processed.

Now return to the two-patient problem with which this chapter opened. Same plan. Same delivery. Different outcomes. The standard framework attributes this to biological variability—the natural spread of radiosensitivity across patients. In that framework, variability is expected to correlate with baseline genomic and microenvironmental features that precede treatment.

What the three anomalies share instead is variability that correlates with the structure of the treatment delivered—with its temporal pattern, its spatial distribution, and its accumulated history across fractions. What is observed is systematic, patterned, and directional—resistance that is calibrated to the specific treatment applied, recurrence that reflects adaptation to a specific policy rather than random escape from it.

These features are not fully accounted for by models in which adaptation arises solely from selection on pre-existing variation (Greaves 2012; Gatenby 2009). Experimental evidence shows that cancer cells can enter treatment-induced, reversible states that alter future response independently of genetic change (Sharma 2010; Shaffer 2017). More recent work demonstrates that gene regulatory networks and even single cells can encode exposure history in ways that modify subsequent behavior, functionally resembling learning (Fernando 2009; Pigozzi 2025; Doan 2026).

Taken together, these findings suggest that response variability may reflect not only pre-existing heterogeneity, but an evolving internal state shaped by the structure and history of treatment. That dependence requires a treatment-responsive state—an internal configuration that evolves with exposure and shapes future response.

The Preface of this book called it the ghost in the cancer. What the next three chapters do is document the evidence for its existence, one axis at a time. What the rest of the book does is give it a body—a formal definition, a set of measurement instruments capable of detecting it, and a treatment architecture capable of acting on what those instruments reveal.

CHAPTER

02

The Temporal Problem

Chapter 1 identified FLASH radiotherapy as the first place where the temporal axis of radiation delivery broke the model's predictions—where delivering the same total dose in a fraction of a second, rather than several minutes, produced a categorically different biological outcome. This chapter examines that break in full: the experimental evidence that established it, the mechanistic explanations that have been proposed and found insufficient, and what the observations imply about the nature of the system being treated. The argument will move from observation to mechanism to necessity—and by the end it will be clear that FLASH is not primarily a story about oxygen or dose rate. It is a story about what kind of thing a tumour is.

In 1956, researchers at the Hammersmith Hospital in London made an observation that should have been unsettling. When they irradiated cells at extremely high dose rates—delivering the same total dose in a fraction of the time normally required—the biological effect was different. Not dramatically, and not yet in a way that commanded sustained attention. But different (Dewey and Boag, 1959).

The observation was filed away. Radiobiology moved forward on the assumption that had served it well for decades: what matters, biologically, is the total dose delivered. The rate of delivery was considered a secondary variable—important in specific contexts like brachytherapy, but generally manageable through repair kinetics and not a fundamental determinant of response.

This assumption held until it didn't.

The Discovery That Restarted the Question

In 2014, a team in France published results that were difficult to dismiss (Favaudon et al., 2014). When radiation was delivered at dose rates exceeding 40 Gray per second—rates orders of magnitude above conventional clinical practice—something unexpected happened. Normal tissue toxicity dropped substantially. Lung damage, the endpoint they were measuring, was dramatically reduced. Tumor control, by contrast, was preserved. The same total dose, delivered in a fraction of a second rather than several minutes, produced a fundamentally different biological outcome.

This differential effect between normal tissue and tumor—normal tissue sparing without loss of tumor kill—is exactly what radiotherapy has always wanted and never reliably achieved. The observation sparked a field. It is now called the FLASH effect, and it has been reproduced across multiple tissue types, multiple species, and multiple irradiation modalities (Vozenin et al., 2019; Montay-Gruel et al., 2017). It is not an artifact. It is real.

What it means, however, has proven far harder to establish than the fact of its existence.

What the Standard Models Predict—and Don't

The linear-quadratic model, the workhorse of clinical radiobiology, makes a specific prediction about dose rate: response should be largely independent of it under most conditions, with some sensitivity arising from repair kinetics during prolonged irradiation (Fowler, 1989). At very high dose rates, where irradiation is complete before significant repair can occur, the model predicts if anything slightly *more* damage, not less. The FLASH observation—dramatically *less* normal tissue damage at ultra-high dose rates—is not merely outside the model's quantitative range. It is in the wrong direction.

This directional wrongness deserves emphasis because it is qualitative, not quantitative. A quantitative failure means the model predicts the right shape but the wrong magnitude—a problem correctable by adjusting parameters. What the FLASH observation produces is something different: the model predicts a flat line, or a slight upward bend, and the data show a threshold followed by a sigmoid rise followed by saturation. These are three features—threshold, sigmoid transition, saturation—that no combination of α and β values can produce from the LQ mathematical structure. The model does not approximate the observation poorly. It is structurally incapable of reproducing it. Figure 2.1 makes this visible directly. The dashed line is not close to the solid line and drifting further. It is a different shape entirely—flat where the data are curved, unconstrained where the data saturate, blind to the threshold that is the observation's most clinically significant feature. When a model fails in this way—not in magnitude but in kind—the appropriate response is not a better fitting procedure. It is a question about what the model is missing.

The most prominent mechanistic explanation invokes radiolytic oxygen depletion (Pratx and Kapp, 2019; Labarbe et al., 2020). At ultra-high dose rates, the argument goes, radiation consumes available oxygen faster than it can be replenished, transiently reducing tissue oxygenation and thereby reducing radiosensitivity. This is physically plausible. But it makes a specific prediction: the sparing effect should scale smoothly and continuously with dose rate, as oxygen depletion increases gradually with delivery speed.

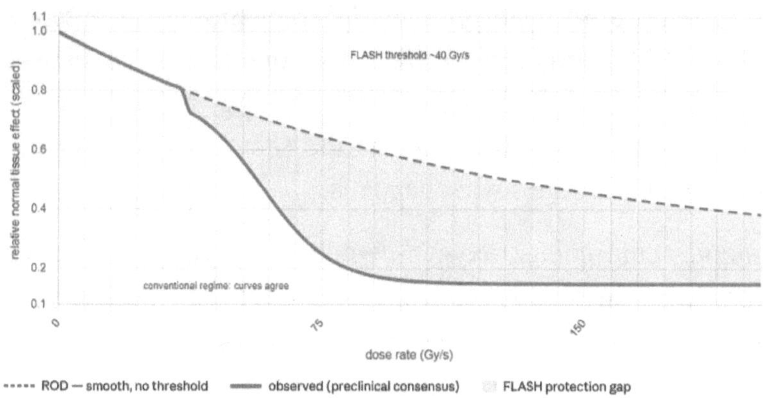

Figure 2.1. *Relative normal tissue effect vs dose rate. ROD predicts a smooth continuous fall with no threshold and no saturation. The observed preclinical consensus shows a flat response below ~40 Gy/s, a sharp accelerated drop above the threshold, and a plateau near 0.15—a 44–58% reduction in damage relative to conventional delivery (Favaudon et al. 2014; Vozenin et al. 2019).*

What is actually observed is different. The FLASH effect has a threshold—below a certain dose rate, essentially nothing happens, and above it, sparing appears sharply (Montay-Gruel et al., 2017; Vozenin et al., 2019). There is also a saturation: beyond a certain dose rate, additional speed does not produce additional sparing. And critically, sparing depends not only on average dose rate but on the fine temporal structure of delivery—the spacing between pulses, the duty cycle, the pattern of how radiation is parceled out over time (Friedl et al., 2022; Vozenin et al., 2019). Two delivery schemes with identical total dose and identical average dose rate can produce different biological outcomes if their pulse structures differ. It is the difference between tapping a glass repeatedly and striking it once with a hammer—the total force can be the same, but the way it is delivered determines what happens.

Smooth, continuous, oxygen-depletion-driven models cannot reproduce threshold behavior, saturation, or sensitivity to pulse structure. Something else is operating.

The System Remembers

The sensitivity to pulse structure is the most conceptually revealing feature of the FLASH effect, and the one that has received insufficient attention.

Consider what pulse-structure sensitivity actually implies. When the spacing between pulses changes the biological outcome—even when total dose and average dose rate are held constant—it means the system's response to any given pulse is influenced by what happened in the preceding pulses. The biological state produced by early pulses modifies how the system responds to later ones. The system is not responding to each pulse independently. It is integrating across time. It has, in the precise dynamical systems sense of the term, memory.

This is the key observation. Not the dose rate per se. Not the oxygen depletion per se. What FLASH is revealing is that the biological system does not respond solely to its current input. It responds to its current input *and* to the state it has been placed in by prior inputs. The path by which a total dose is delivered—not merely the destination—determines the outcome.

This conclusion has been formalized in the M-ROD framework (see Appendix A and B), which extends classical radiolytic oxygen depletion by coupling it to a bounded, history-dependent internal state variable. The internal state activates nonlinearly above a dose rate threshold, reinforces itself through feedback, decays between pulses, and saturates at high activation. This minimal architecture—whose dynamics are consistent with those of cooperative biological regulatory processes including gene regulatory networks—reproduces threshold behavior, saturation, pulse-spacing dependence, and time-ordering sensitivity simultaneously. The classical oxygen-depletion model is recovered as a limiting case when the internal state is inactive. The full mathematical derivation is given in Appendix A.

What this demonstrates—as a proof of concept, pending independent experimental validation—is that a system with an evolving internal state can produce all the features of FLASH that memoryless models cannot. The implication is not that M-ROD is the final model. It is that *some* internal state must exist. The data demand it.

The Order of Delivery Matters

One experimental signature deserves particular emphasis because its implications are rarely stated explicitly. When radiation is delivered in two phases—one at high dose rate followed by one at low dose rate, versus the reverse sequence—the biological outcome differs, even though the total dose and the dose rates used are identical in both cases (Appendix B).

This is a remarkable result. It means that the biological effect of a radiation treatment is not determined solely by what doses were delivered and at what rates. It is also determined by *when* each component was applied—by the order of events in time.

In physics, order matters when a system has state. A ball rolling on a flat surface reaches the same position regardless of the path taken. A ball rolling on a landscape with hills and valleys reaches different positions depending on the path—because its trajectory is shaped by the terrain it has already traversed. FLASH is telling us that the biological landscape is the second kind. The tumor is a system with terrain. Its response to any intervention depends on where it is in that landscape at the moment of intervention, and where it is depends on the history of prior interventions.

This is not a minor technical complication. It is a fundamental statement about the nature of the system being treated. A system whose response depends on the order of its inputs cannot be fully described by any model that treats each input independently. The system has an internal configuration—a state—that evolves over time and shapes what each new input does.

What the Temporal Problem Tells Us

FLASH radiotherapy is not primarily a story about oxygen. It is a story about time and memory. The observations reveal a system that integrates its experience—that carries its past forward into its present behavior in ways that cannot be captured by models that see only the current input.

The conventional radiobiological framework is memoryless by construction: dose accumulates, damage accumulates, but the system itself has no evolving internal configuration that shapes its sensitivity to future inputs. FLASH shows that this construction is incomplete. The system remembers. And what it remembers changes what we can do to it.

What FLASH has established is not a new mechanism to be added to the model. It is structural evidence that the system has an inside—an internal state that integrates prior exposure and shapes how each subsequent fraction is processed, independently of what total accumulated dose predicts. Chapter 1 called this the ghost in the cancer. FLASH is the first place it becomes visible. The temporal axis of radiation delivery, pushed beyond the range conventional fractionation ever explored, has exposed a history-dependence that no parameter adjustment within the existing framework can accommodate. The state exists. The temporal data demand it.

Now, we need to ask whether a similar failure appears not in time but in space—whether the assumption that different regions of a tumor behave independently is equally unsound.

That is the question the next chapter addresses.

CHAPTER

03

The Spatial Problem

Chapter 1 identified SFRT as the second place where radiation delivery broke the model's predictions—where leaving large portions of the tumour deliberately unirradiated produced responses that uniform delivery could not match, and where unirradiated regions responded as though they had been treated. This chapter examines that break in full: the experimental evidence, the mechanistic explanations proposed and found structurally insufficient, and what the spatial pattern of response reveals about the kind of system a tumour actually is.

Radiotherapy has always known that tumors are not uniform. Imaging makes this visible—regions of high and low density, areas of necrosis surrounded by viable tissue, gradients of oxygenation that vary across millimeters. The biological heterogeneity of tumors is not a secret. It is one of the central challenges of treatment planning.

And yet, the standard radiobiological framework treats this heterogeneity in a specific way: each region of the tumor responds according to its local properties. Different radiosensitivity, different oxygenation, different repair capacity—these differences are acknowledged and modeled. What is not modeled, as a default, is the *relationship* between regions. The assumption is that each part of the tumor responds to the radiation it receives, independently of what is happening elsewhere.

This assumption has a name in mathematics: it is the assumption of spatial independence. And like the assumption of temporal memorylessness examined in the previous chapter, it has begun to fail under the pressure of observation.

The Evidence From an Unlikely Technique

The clearest experimental challenge to spatial independence comes from one of the oldest and most counterintuitive techniques in radiation oncology: spatially fractionated radiotherapy, or SFRT.

The basic idea of SFRT is deliberately provocative. Instead of delivering dose uniformly across the tumor—which decades of conventional planning have optimized—SFRT delivers radiation in a highly non-uniform pattern. Using grid or lattice arrangements, high-dose regions are interspersed with regions of low or essentially zero dose. A substantial portion of the tumor volume is, by design, left undertreated in any given fraction.

By the logic of spatial independence, this should be counterproductive. Untreated regions should continue growing unimpeded. The net effect should be inferior to uniform irradiation of the same total dose. The partial treatment of the tumor should produce partial control at best.

This is not what happens.

Before examining the evidence, the nature of the failure deserves to be stated precisely. The spatial independence assumption embedded in the LQ model is not an approximation that degrades gracefully as coupling increases. It is binary. Either each region responds only to its own local dose, or it does not. Any measurable response in an unirradiated valley region—however small, however mediated—falsifies the assumption completely. There is no parameter adjustment within the existing framework that can produce a valley response from a model that assumes independence. The failure, when it comes, will not be quantitative. It will be categorical.

SFRT has demonstrated effective tumor control—in some cases striking control—for large, bulky tumors that respond poorly to conventional uniform irradiation (Mohiuddin et al., 1999; Griffin et al., 2020). The untreated regions do not simply continue growing as though the treatment did not occur. Something propagates from the irradiated regions to their neighbors. The response is not local. It is systemic within the tumor. It is less like treating isolated patches of tissue and more like pulling on one part of a spider web—the entire structure shifts, including regions you never touched directly.

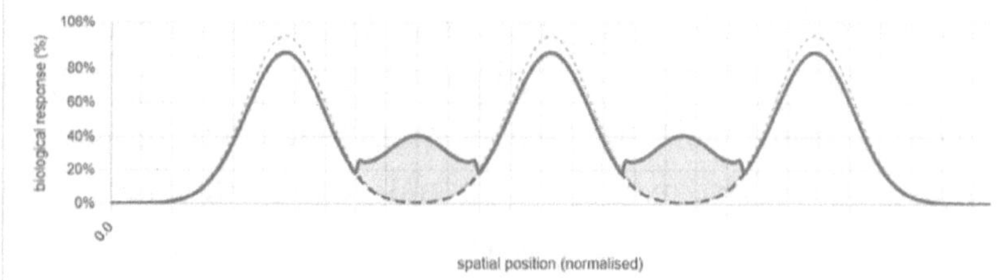

Figure 3.1: *Spatial response heterogeneity in SFRT: deviation from LQ prediction.Observed biological response (solid line) across normalized spatial position shows nonlocal effects extending beyond high-dose regions, deviating from the locally dose-dependent prediction of the Linear–Quadratic model (dashed line).*

The Mechanisms Proposed—and Their Shared Limitation

Several mechanisms have been proposed to explain how irradiated regions influence non-irradiated ones. Bystander effects—the well-documented phenomenon whereby irradiated cells release signals that alter the behavior of neighboring non-irradiated cells—are one candidate (Prise and O'Sullivan, 2009). Immune-mediated responses, in which radiation-induced cell death triggers local and sometimes systemic immune activation, are another (Demaria and Formenti, 2015). Vascular effects, through which radiation alters blood supply and microenvironmental conditions across a wider spatial domain than the directly irradiated volume, have also been invoked (Garcia-Barros et al., 2003).

Each of these mechanisms is real. Each contributes something to the explanation. But taken together, they share a structural limitation that mirrors what we saw with the mechanistic explanations for FLASH. They are descriptive accounts of how influence might propagate—they do not provide a predictive framework for *how much* influence will propagate, in what direction, over what spatial scale, and under what delivery conditions. Each mechanism is introduced to explain a specific observation. None generalizes naturally to the full pattern of SFRT results.

There is one further phenomenon that sharpens this structural limitation into clinical visibility. The abscopal effect—regression of tumors at sites entirely distant from the irradiated field, documented across multiple tumor types (Grass et al., 2016; Reynders et al., 2019)—is the organizational coupling argument made visible at its most extreme. It is not a neighboring region responding to what happens in an irradiated region. It is a metastatic site, separated by centimeters or meters of unirradiated tissue, responding to a perturbation delivered elsewhere entirely. No local model can accommodate this. No sum of independent regional responses produces it. It is the clinical signature of a system whose response is governed by something distributed across the whole—an organizational state that propagates consequences far beyond the volume that received the dose. That it occurs unpredictably, in some patients and not others with no reliable baseline predictor, is not a curiosity. It is precisely the fingerprint of a hidden organizational state that current measurements cannot characterize.

The deeper problem is that these mechanisms are all framed as additions to a fundamentally local model. The base assumption—that each region responds primarily to its own irradiation—remains intact, with non-local effects treated as secondary corrections. But if regions are genuinely coupled, if information propagates across the tumor as a fundamental feature of its dynamics rather than as a secondary perturbation, then a local model with corrections is the wrong starting point. The right starting point is a system.

What Coupling Actually Means

A tumor that behaves as a coupled spatial system is one in which the state of any region depends not only on its own history and inputs, but on the states of its neighbors. Vascularization creates shared microenvironments. Gap junctions and signaling molecules create channels for intercellular communication. The immune microenvironment responds to signals from multiple regions simultaneously. Mechanical stresses generated by growth and treatment propagate across tissue boundaries (Jain, 1987; Gatenby and Gillies, 2009; Osswald et al., 2015).

In such a system, delivering dose to one region is not only an intervention on that region. It is a perturbation to a network—one that will propagate through the network's connections and produce effects that extend beyond the directly treated volume. The spatial distribution of dose is not merely a geometric question of coverage. It is a question of how perturbations propagate through a coupled dynamical system.

This reframing has a precise mathematical consequence that is worth stating explicitly, because it reveals a fundamental limitation of standard clinical metrics. In a spatially coupled system, the mean response across the tumor—the average of what all regions are doing—is mathematically insensitive to the coupling between them. The coupling terms cancel when you take the average, leaving the mean trajectory indistinguishable from what an independent system would produce (see Appendix A and B). Two tumors—one with strong spatial coupling between its regions, one with none—can produce identical mean ADC trajectories on serial MRI scans, even though their internal dynamics are completely different.

This is not a measurement problem. It is a structural property of how averages work in coupled systems. Standard imaging metrics, built around scalar summaries of tumor response, are blind to the coupling that may be one of the most clinically important features of the system.

This is precisely what the TCI framework was designed to address (Appendix A and B). Rather than measuring average response, TCI measures predictive improvement: does knowing the state of a tumor region's neighbors improve prediction of its future state? If the spatial model predicts better than the independent model, structure exists. The coupling is real, even if invisible to conventional metrics. The full theoretical development of TCI and its integration into the informational state framework is given in Appendix A.

The Failure of Additivity

There is a related assumption embedded in most radiobiological planning that SFRT puts under pressure: the assumption that effects are additive across space. The biological effect of a dose distribution should, on this view, be predictable from the sum of its local contributions. High-dose regions contribute their effect; low-dose regions contribute theirs; the overall outcome is the weighted aggregate.

SFRT violates this. The outcome is not the weighted sum of local responses. The spatial *arrangement* of high- and low-dose regions—which regions are neighbors, how the pattern is oriented, how the gradients are structured—influences the outcome in ways that pure additivity cannot capture (Zhang et al., 2020). The system responds to its configuration, not merely to the magnitude of its inputs summed across space.

This failure of additivity is the spatial analogue of the failure of temporal independence we saw in FLASH. There, response depended on the order and spacing of inputs in time. Here, response depends on the arrangement and connectivity of inputs in space. In both cases, what breaks down is the assumption that the system can be decomposed into independent parts whose contributions can simply be added together.

A system that cannot be decomposed in time, and cannot be decomposed in space, is a system with genuine internal structure—one in which parts interact to produce collective behavior that cannot be read off from the parts individually.

A Hint About What the Tumor Is

The spatial problem points toward something that will become central in Part II of this book. A tumor that responds to spatial patterns of irradiation—that propagates effects between regions, that cannot be described by local models even when each region is individually well-characterized—is not a collection of independent units that happen to be located near each other. It is a *system* in the meaningful sense: an entity defined by the relationships between its parts as much as by the parts themselves.

In such systems, the relevant question is not only what each region contains—what cells, what mutations, what oxygenation level—but how the regions are connected, how information flows between them, and what organizational properties govern the collective behavior. The tumor has spatial structure that is causally relevant. That structure shapes how interventions propagate. And that structure is, at present, almost entirely unmeasured in clinical practice.

There is a further implication that connects directly to what Chapter 1 called the ghost—the hidden internal configuration of the tumour that the model cannot see and that determines which trajectory the system follows under treatment pressure. If the tumor is a coupled spatial system, then the information content of a spatially structured treatment—a grid pattern, a lattice arrangement—is very different from the information content of uniform irradiation. SFRT does not simply deliver dose. It perturbs the network. And a network that processes information about perturbations—that uses the spatial pattern of stress to infer something about the threat and reorganize accordingly—will respond differently to different spatial patterns. Resistance, in this light, is not only temporal adaptation to repeated exposure. It is also spatial reorganization in response to spatially structured pressure.

The tumor learns from the pattern, not just the magnitude.

Toward the Third Axis

The spatial problem adds a second dimension to what is becoming a consistent pattern. The temporal problem showed that the *when* of irradiation matters in ways that memoryless models cannot capture. The spatial problem shows that the *where* matters in ways that independent models cannot capture. Both failures point to the same underlying reality: the system has internal structure—temporal memory, spatial coupling—that conventional models do not represent. The response to radiation is not a local, instantaneous function of local, instantaneous dose. It is a property of the system's full configuration in space and time.

What SFRT has established structurally mirrors what FLASH established in the previous chapter, but along a different axis. FLASH showed that the system carries its temporal experience forward—that the state the system is in at the moment of any pulse depends on what preceded it. SFRT shows that the system carries its spatial organisation forward—that the state of any region is not independent of the states of its neighbours, and that perturbations propagate through the organisational structure of the whole in ways that no local model can reproduce. In both cases what is revealed is the same thing: the tumour has an inside. A distributed internal configuration that is not captured by any measurement of individual components, that evolves under the pressure of treatment, and that governs what each new intervention encounters. Chapter 1 named this the ghost. The temporal axis made it visible in time. The spatial axis has now made it visible in space. One more axis remains.

Even if we set aside temporal structure entirely, and deliver dose uniformly across space at conventional rates, the relationship between dose and response begins to break down in a third and equally fundamental way—when the dose itself becomes very large.

That failure is the subject of the next chapter.

CHAPTER

04

The High-Dose Problem: When More Stops Meaning More

Chapter 1 identified SBRT as the third place where radiation delivery broke the model's predictions—where pushing dose per fraction beyond a certain threshold produced outcomes that the LQ model could not reliably predict and that its extensions could not consistently reconcile. This chapter examines that break in full. It begins with the clinical logic that made dose escalation irresistible, then shows precisely where and how that logic runs out.

There is a seductive logic to dose escalation in radiotherapy. If radiation kills cancer cells, then more radiation should kill more cancer cells. If a tumor recurs after treatment, perhaps the dose was insufficient. If outcomes are variable, perhaps the solution is to push harder. The history of radiotherapy contains many chapters written in this spirit—progressive escalation of dose, driven by the belief that the relationship between dose and tumor control is fundamentally one of more is better.

Stereotactic Body Radiotherapy represents the most dramatic modern expression of this logic. By concentrating treatment into a small number of fractions—sometimes as few as three to five—each delivering doses per fraction that conventional fractionation would never attempt, SBRT achieves local control rates in some tumor types that are genuinely impressive. For early-stage lung cancer, for liver metastases, for spinal tumors, the results have been striking enough to shift clinical practice substantially (Timmerman et al., 2010; Potters et al., 2004).

And yet, the closer you look at what SBRT is doing biologically, the more the underlying theory begins to fray.

The Model That Was Never Designed for This

The linear-quadratic model was validated within a specific domain—modest doses per fraction, conventional delivery rates, fractionated treatment with time for repair between sessions (Fowler, 1989). Within that domain it is reliable. The question SBRT poses is what happens when that domain is systematically exceeded.

When SBRT arrived and began delivering doses per fraction of 10, 15, 20 Gray or more, the temptation was to simply extend the LQ model into this new regime. The mathematics permitted it. The biology, as it turned out, did not.

At high doses per fraction, the LQ model predicts cell killing that grows increasingly rapidly with dose—the quadratic term dominates, and the survival curve bends steeply downward.

This prediction has been shown to overestimate actual cell killing at very high doses in multiple experimental systems (Astrahan, 2008; Kirkpatrick et al., 2008). The model, extrapolated beyond its domain of validity, becomes unreliable in the direction of overclaiming—predicting more damage than actually occurs.

This matters beyond the quantitative error. Figure 4.1 makes the geometry of the failure visible. Below approximately 8 Gy per fraction the two curves track together—the model is adequate in its designed domain. Above that threshold the observed survival curve straightens into a log-linear relationship while the LQ curve continues bending steeply downward. These are not two curves that are close and drifting apart. They are two curves with different shapes—one continuously curving, one transitioning to linear. No adjustment of α or β changes the shape of the LQ prediction. The quadratic term forces continuous curvature regardless of parameter values. What Figure 4.1 shows is therefore not a quantitative failure correctable by better fitting. It is a regime boundary—a point beyond which the mathematical structure of the model is no longer compatible with what the biology is doing.

The practical consequences are significant. The biologically effective dose, or BED—the clinical tool derived from the LQ model that allows comparison of different fractionation schemes—becomes mathematically unstable at high doses per fraction. Small changes in the assumed alpha/beta ratio produce large changes in predicted BED. Different extensions of the model—the LQ-linear formulation, the universal survival curve—make divergent predictions for the same physical dose (Park et al., 2008; Guerrero and Li, 2004). The quantitative foundation for comparing SBRT regimens with each other, or with conventional fractionation, becomes genuinely uncertain precisely where clinical decision-making most needs it to be reliable.

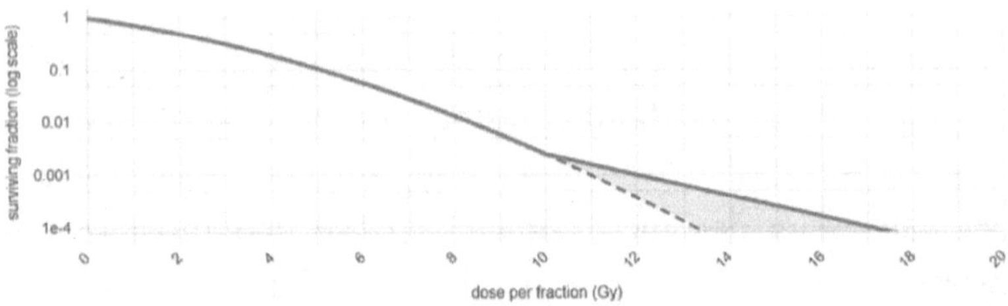

Figure 4.1: *Deviation from Linear–Quadratic prediction at high dose per fraction (SBRT regime). At low-to-moderate doses, observed cell survival (solid line) follows the Linear–Quadratic model (dashed line). At high doses per fraction, a systematic deviation emerges, indicating breakdown of LQ assumptions and the contribution of additional biological effects not captured by the model*

The Variability That Dose Cannot Explain

Beyond the theoretical instability, there is a clinical observation that deserves more attention than it typically receives. Patients receiving SBRT for similar tumors, under similar regimens, with similarly precise delivery, show outcomes that vary more than a dose-based model predicts they should.

If biological response were primarily determined by the physical dose delivered, and if delivery is highly accurate and reproducible—which modern SBRT systems genuinely achieve—then outcome variability should be modest and attributable to known sources: patient anatomy, tumor histology, intrinsic radiosensitivity as characterized by standard parameters. What is observed instead is a wider spread of outcomes than these factors explain (Fowler, 2010). Some tumors respond dramatically to doses that produce minimal effect in apparently similar cases. Others recur quickly despite receiving doses that should, by the model, produce durable control.

This residual variability is often discussed in terms of biological factors not captured by current models—immune response, vascular effects, microenvironmental conditions. And these contributions are real. But the pattern of variability itself—its persistence across tumor types and treatment centers, its resistance to explanation by known measurable factors—suggests that something more fundamental is at work. The system's response to a large dose is not determined solely by the dose and the few variables currently measured. Something about the system's condition at the time of treatment—the hidden internal configuration that Chapter 1 called the ghost—is contributing to the outcome in ways that dose alone cannot capture and that current measurements do not track.

What High Doses Actually Do

Several mechanisms have been proposed to explain why very high doses per fraction produce effects that go beyond what simple cell killing predicts. Vascular damage—the direct destruction of tumor blood vessels at high doses, leading to indirect tumor cell death through loss of support—has substantial experimental backing (Garcia-Barros et al., 2003). Immune activation—the release of tumor antigens from radiation-killed cells, triggering systemic immune responses that contribute to local and sometimes distant control—has generated considerable interest, including through the phenomenon of the abscopal effect (Demaria and Formenti, 2015). Endothelial apoptosis and disruption of stromal support have also been identified as components of high-dose response not captured by clonogenic cell killing models alone.

These mechanisms are genuine. But taken together, they illustrate the same structural problem we have encountered repeatedly. Each mechanism was proposed to explain a specific observation. Each operates differently, involves different cell populations and signaling pathways, and dominates under different conditions. No unified framework integrates them into a coherent, predictive description of high-dose response. The result is a collection of post-hoc explanations—added to the model after the observation is made, not derived from a framework that predicted it in advance.

This is the signature of a model operating at its boundaries. When a theory can only explain its anomalies by adding new mechanisms case by case, the anomalies are telling you something the theory's structure cannot accommodate. They are not exceptions to the rule. They are signals that the rule is incomplete.

A Regime Change, Not a Scaling Failure

The most honest interpretation of what SBRT reveals is not that the LQ model needs a better correction factor at high doses. It is that high doses per fraction push the biological system into a qualitatively different regime—one governed by dynamics that the LQ model, by construction, cannot represent. It is like increasing the load on a structure: up to a point, it deforms in proportion to the force applied; beyond that point, it no longer deforms—it fails.

In dynamical systems, this kind of qualitative shift has a name: a regime transition, or in some contexts, a phase transition. Systems that behave one way under small perturbations can behave in a fundamentally different way under large ones—not because the rules change, but because the large perturbation drives the system across a threshold into a region of state space with different stability properties. The system is not doing more of the same thing. It is doing something different.

There is growing evidence that biological systems, including tumor systems, exhibit this kind of threshold behavior. Gene regulatory networks switch between stable states rather than varying continuously (Tyson and Novak, 2010). Cellular populations can undergo rapid transitions in phenotype under sufficient stress (Gatenby and Gillies, 2009). The resistance patterns observed after SBRT—often qualitatively different from those following conventional fractionation, occurring faster and in different forms—are more consistent with state transitions than with smooth dose-response scaling.

If this interpretation is correct, then the SBRT variability problem is not noise to be reduced by better delivery precision. It is the signature of a system whose response to large perturbations depends on its internal state at the moment of perturbation—on which region of its state space it currently occupies, and therefore which trajectory the perturbation will initiate. Two tumors receiving identical doses can follow entirely different trajectories not because of measurement error but because they were in different states when treated. States that current measurements do not capture.

CHAPTER

05

A Pattern in the Failures

The three preceding chapters told three different stories. A physicist working on radiation delivery would recognise them as separate technical problems—one about dose rate, one about spatial distribution, one about dose magnitude. They involve different machine parameters, different biological mechanisms proposed to explain them, and different research communities working on them.

And yet something nags.

When you step back from the individual cases and look at all three together, a discomfort sets in. The failures are too consistent, too symmetrically distributed, to be coincidence. FLASH breaks the model along the axis of time. SFRT breaks it along the axis of space. SBRT breaks it along the axis of magnitude. These are not three anomalies. They are one pattern, visible from three different angles.

This chapter names that pattern—and follows it to its necessary conclusion.

Three Axes, One Failure Mode

Radiation can only be varied along three fundamental dimensions: when it is delivered, where it is delivered, and how much is delivered. Time, space, and magnitude. There is no fourth axis.

In each case, the existing model makes a specific simplifying assumption—memorylessness in time, spatial independence, continuous dose-response scaling—and in each case that assumption breaks down under conditions that push the relevant dimension to its extremes. The breakdown is not a smooth degradation of accuracy. It is a qualitative failure: thresholds where there should be gradients, non-local effects where there should be local independence, regime transitions where there should be proportional scaling (Favaudon et al., 2014; Vozenin et al., 2019; Mohiuddin et al., 1999; Griffin et al., 2020; Fowler, 2010; Kirkpatrick et al., 2008).

Three assumptions. Three failures. Three axes. The symmetry is not accidental.

What the Failures Share

Look past the surface differences and a single feature unites all three: in each case, response depends on context in a way that the existing model cannot represent. Context here means something precise—not merely background conditions, but the internal configuration of the system at the moment of irradiation, shaped by its history, its spatial organisation, and its current dynamical state.

The conventional model has no representation of any of this. It maps inputs to outputs through fixed relationships, treating the system as though it has no internal structure beyond its measurable variables. It is, in the language of dynamical systems theory, a memoryless input-output map—and memoryless maps cannot produce the behaviours observed (Bellman and Åström, 1970; Villaverde et al., 2016). The failure of decomposability this represents—the impossibility of predicting the whole from the independent sum of its parts—is the defining property of complex dynamical systems, and the tumour is a canonical example of it (Kitano, 2002; Tyson and Novak, 2010).

This is not a criticism of the LQ model as such. For the conditions under which it was designed—modest doses, conventional fractionation, spatially homogeneous delivery—it remains a useful approximation. The criticism is of its extension beyond those conditions without recognising that a qualitative boundary has been crossed.

The Signal

There is a precise way to describe what these failures are pointing to. In each case, the system's response cannot be determined from the input alone. Something else is necessary—some description of the system's internal condition at the time of irradiation. That internal condition evolves over time, reflects the history of prior exposures, and constrains which behaviours are currently accessible. It is not directly observable. But its influence is pervasive.

This is the first clear signature of what we have called the ghost in the cancer.

Not a metaphor. A structural consequence. Any system exhibiting history-dependence, spatial coupling, and nonlinear regime transitions can be modelled either by introducing an internal state that carries those properties or by expanding the input space to include every variable whose history would matter—and in practice, for biological systems of this complexity, the state-based formulation is the tractable choice (Kalman, 1960; Friston et al., 2017). The anomalies are not anomalies under either formulation. They are the fingerprints of structure that the classical framework—which assumes memorylessness, spatial independence, and continuous dose scaling—has no variable to represent.

A Different Kind of Problem

This recognition changes what radiotherapy is, as a problem.

If tumour response is state-dependent, then the central question is no longer simply what dose to deliver. It is what state the system is in—and what actions, across time, space, and magnitude, will guide that state toward a desired trajectory. This is a fundamentally different kind of problem. It is not an optimisation problem over a dose distribution. It is a control problem over a partially observable dynamical system (Kaelbling et al., 1998).

There is a further implication that will become important later. Tumours do not merely have hidden states—they adapt. Clonal populations compete. Resistant subpopulations emerge under treatment pressure not randomly, but in response to the selective environment that treatment creates (Gatenby et al., 2009; Zhang et al., 2017). This means that the tumour is not a passive system being acted upon. It is, in a meaningful evolutionary sense, a strategic system—one that responds to the policy the clinician applies with adaptive counter-moves. The key finding—that driving sensitive populations to extinction can accelerate resistance by removing competitive suppression of resistant clones—suggests that the optimal treatment policy must anticipate the tumour's evolutionary response, not merely optimise against its current state (Gatenby and Brown, 2020).

All of this is downstream of the pattern identified in this chapter. FLASH, SFRT, and SBRT are the first evidence. The rest of the book builds the response.

From Pattern to Framework

The next step is not to propose another mechanistic explanation for each anomaly separately. That approach has already been tried—and has produced a proliferation of competing, context-specific models, none of which generalise—and none of which, even among the state-based formulations discussed in Chapter 6, addresses the regimes Part I has documented, and all of which share the structural limitation identified here (Chis et al., 2011; Villaverde et al., 2016).

From Pattern to Framework

The next step is not to propose another mechanistic explanation for each anomaly separately. That approach has already been tried—and has produced a proliferation of competing, context-specific models, none of which generalise, all of which share the structural limitation identified here (Chis et al., 2011; Villaverde et al., 2016). Part II builds the language the conventional framework lacks—beginning not with equations, but with biology: with the question of what kind of thing a tumour actually is, and what properties it must have to produce the behaviours we have now documented.

The ghost has been seen from three angles. It is time to understand what it is.

PART II

From Biology to Information

The five chapters that follow are the most demanding in the book. They move from the failure of mechanistic explanation, through the biology of networked systems and memory, to the formal definition of the informational state and its physical instantiation in living tissue. This is not background material. It is the foundation on which the measurement instruments of Part III and the treatment architecture of Part IV are built. Without it, the framework has no ground to stand on.

The clinician reader who followed the clinical spine—Preface, Chapters 1 through 5—is invited to continue directly to Chapter 11, where the six rules summarize what Part II establishes. But something will be lost in that jump: the biological reality that makes the rules more than assertions, and the physical necessity that makes the informational state more than a convenient abstraction. Part II is where the ghost gets a body. It rewards the reader who stays with it.

For those who continue: the density is intentional. Each chapter builds on the previous one. Chapter 9 in particular—the informational state and top-down causation—is the conceptual core of the entire framework. It is worth reading slowly.

CHAPTER

06

Why Mechanistic Understanding Is Not Enough

Chapter 5 established that the classical radiobiological framework is inadequate to the observational record, and that a unified response to that inadequacy points toward a framework organised around a hidden internal state. The question this chapter addresses is a different one: why cannot adding more mechanistic detail to the existing framework substitute for representing that state directly?

The answer—the identifiability problem—is the structural reason why the mechanistic research programme, however rich, cannot close the gap that Part I documented.

The Appeal of More Detail

Modern biology has achieved something remarkable. The molecular machinery of DNA damage and repair is described in extraordinary detail (Jeggo and Löbrich, 2007). Signaling pathways that govern cell survival and death are mapped with increasing completeness (Hanahan and Weinberg, 2011). The tumor microenvironment—the ecosystem of immune cells, fibroblasts, vasculature, and extracellular matrix that surrounds and infiltrates the tumor—is recognized as a crucial determinant of behavior (Junttila and de Sauvage, 2013). The interactions between radiation and each of these components have been studied extensively.

Given this, the mechanistic research program has a clear logic. If conventional radiobiology misses the mark because its models are too simple, then the solution is richer models—ones that capture more of the biology we now understand. More pathways. More variables. More detail.

This logic is not wrong in principle. But it collides, in practice, with a problem that more detail cannot solve.

A Parallel Lineage: Internal-State Models Already in Radiobiology

Before turning to the identifiability problem, it is worth acknowledging that internal-state formulations are not new to radiobiology. The Lethal-Potentially Lethal model of Curtis (1986) introduced two populations of lesions—repairable and irreparable—whose evolution under competing first- and second-order kinetics carries irradiation history forward and shapes subsequent response. The Repair-Misrepair formulation of Tobias (1985) tracks lesion populations as they evolve between correct repair and misrepair. The saturable-repair models in the tradition of Goodhead (1985) introduce finite repair-enzyme pools whose depletion under high damage loads produces threshold-like behaviour in cell survival. The Microdosimetric Kinetic Model of Hawkins (1994, 2003) tracks sublesion populations in subcellular domains with explicit dynamics and has been developed into the basis for much of modern ion-therapy treatment planning. The Local Effect Model of Scholz and Kraft (1996) reconstructs biological effect from spatial distributions of track-induced lesions and is used clinically in European carbon-ion centres.

Each of these is, in a precise sense, an internal-state model. Each introduces a variable—a lesion population, a repair-enzyme pool, a sublesion count—whose current value carries the influence of prior irradiation forward and determines response to the next increment of dose. The framework developed in this book is therefore not the first to treat radiobiology as requiring state-based description. What distinguishes it from these earlier formulations is not the idea of hidden internal dynamics—which the field has had for forty years—but three specific commitments: the proposal of a distributed, organisational state rather than a population of lesions; the identification of that state with bioelectric organisational memory drawing on experimental work in model organisms (Chapter 10); and the application to the specific regimes of FLASH, SFRT, and SBRT, which the earlier formulations were not designed to address and which lie outside their domain of validity. The prior models remain useful within their domains. The framework proposed here extends state-based thinking into regimes where those domains no longer hold.

The Identifiability Problem

In 1949, the economist Tjalling Koopmans formalized a question that cuts across every field that builds models from data: when can the internal structure of a system be uniquely determined from its observable outputs? He called this the identification problem (Koopmans, 1949). The answer, in general, is unsettling: often it cannot. Multiple different internal configurations—different combinations of parameter values, different causal structures—can produce identical observable behavior. No amount of data can distinguish between them, because they are observationally equivalent.

This is not a statistical problem, solvable with larger samples or better measurement. It is a structural property of the relationship between the system's internal configuration and what it makes visible from the outside. Koopmans recognized it in economic models. Thomas Sargent later demonstrated it with particular force in macroeconomics, showing that competing theories of monetary policy—theories with fundamentally different causal structures—could produce identical predictions for observable economic data, making them impossible to distinguish from observation alone (Sargent, 1976). The identification problem, in this context, was not a failure of measurement. It was a property of what the data could and could not reveal about the underlying system.

The same problem appears with equal force in biological systems. In systems biology, structural identifiability—the question of whether a model's parameters can in principle be uniquely determined from measurable outputs—has been studied formally and found to be deeply problematic for nonlinear dynamic models of even moderate complexity (Chis et al., 2011; Villaverde et al., 2016). Gene regulatory networks with different connectivity can produce the same expression dynamics. Signaling pathways with different rate constants can produce the same downstream outputs. Two tumors with different internal configurations can look identical under every measurement we routinely take.

This is the identifiability problem in biological systems, and it has a direct clinical consequence. If different internal configurations produce the same observable behavior, then observing the behavior—however precisely—cannot tell you which configuration you are dealing with. And if you cannot determine the configuration, you cannot reliably predict how the system will respond to interventions that depend on that configuration.

But the identifiability problem is doing something stronger than establishing a limitation on prediction. It is establishing the existence of the hidden state itself.

The logical structure is precise. In the years since FLASH, SFRT, and SBRT each generated anomalies that conventional radiobiology could not explain, the community has responded in the way science normally responds: by adding more mechanisms, more parameters, and more measurable variables. And yet prediction has remained unreliable. The residual variability has not diminished in proportion to the biological detail added. Despite increasingly detailed mechanistic understanding, predictive performance at the individual level remains limited.

This is not what should happen if the problem is merely one of insufficient mechanistic knowledge. It is exactly what should happen if the system possesses internal states that are not recoverable from observable outputs regardless of how many additional mechanisms are measured and modeled. A system whose observable outputs are consistent with multiple distinct internal configurations simultaneously cannot be uniquely characterized by any finite set of observations. The hidden state is not introduced as a theoretical convenience. It is the most parsimonious response to the observed pattern of failures—more parsimonious than modality-specific mechanistic patches, and more tractable than expanding the input space to every variable whose history might matter.

A more formally systems-theoretic treatment of this argument has been developed separately by me through structural identifiability analysis of representative mechanistic models from FLASH, SFRT, SBRT, and adaptive resistance dynamics (Vaitheeswaran, 2026c). That work analyzed the Pratx-Kapp radiolytic oxygen depletion model for FLASH radiotherapy, the McMahon kinetic-bystander signalling model for SFRT, the LQ-L extension used in SBRT, and the Gupta phenotypic-plasticity model of adaptive resistance. Using generating-series identifiability analysis, Lie-derivative tableaus, symmetry analysis, Jacobian rank evaluation, singular-value decomposition, and profile-likelihood methods, the study examined whether the mechanistic parameters and internal state structure of these models could be uniquely recovered from the observation regimes typically available in radiotherapy experiments and clinical practice.

The results revealed two distinct forms of identifiability failure. The Pratx-Kapp and McMahon models exhibited intrinsic non-identifiability under conventional surviving-fraction observation, where very different internal parameter configurations produced indistinguishable observable dose-response behavior. In the Pratx-Kapp model, for example, doubling the oxygen depletion parameter while halving the oxygen-curvature parameter and rescaling baseline oxygen tension produced exactly the same surviving-fraction curves despite very different hidden oxygen trajectories during irradiation. The LQ-L and Gupta models revealed a complementary problem: recoverability depended directly on how much of the system was being observed. In SBRT, observing only high-dose outcomes collapsed multiple parameter combinations into the same response, whereas including both low-dose and high-dose measurements restored identifiability. In adaptive-resistance studies, single-marker observations made distinct transition dynamics appear identical, while multi-marker longitudinal measurements separated them. Across all four regimes, the analyses repeatedly suggested that clinically observable response may represent only a compressed projection of a richer evolving internal tumor organization.

The implication is not that the underlying biological mechanisms are false. Oxygen depletion, bystander signalling, vascular response, and phenotypic plasticity may all be biologically real processes. The deeper issue is that the same observable outcome may be compatible with multiple distinct internal system organizations. A useful analogy is estimating the economic activity of a city at night using only satellite images of its light patterns. Similar visible light distributions may arise from fundamentally different underlying realities—a wealthy but sparsely populated coastal city, a densely crowded manufacturing hub operating through the night, a city experiencing a large public festival, or a region under emergency power concentration after an infrastructure failure. From high altitude, these very different internal conditions may generate remarkably similar observable light signatures. The observation contains information, but it does not uniquely specify the hidden organizational structure generating it. In such a setting, attempting to recover one exact underlying configuration from a single observation is often less useful than maintaining probabilistic beliefs over multiple plausible explanations and continuously refining those beliefs as additional observations become available over time.

The same logic applies under partial observability in radiobiology. If distinct internal tumor organizations can generate similar observable treatment responses, then prediction and control are improved not by committing to a single recovered parameter set, but by operating adaptively over a distribution of possible underlying states and updating that distribution as treatment-generated observations accumulate. The value of an inference-based framework in such settings is therefore not that it eliminates uncertainty, but that it provides a principled way to operate under uncertainty when the hidden organizational state cannot be uniquely reconstructed from observable measurements alone.

This move—from observed input-output failure to the existence of a hidden internal state—has been made explicitly across five independent fields, each time transforming the discipline. In macroeconomics, Lucas (1976) demonstrated that ignoring the hidden states of economic agents—their expectations and beliefs—produces systematic, predictable policy failures, a conclusion recognized by the Nobel Prize in 1995. In control engineering, Kalman (1960) established that non-observability is not a measurement problem but a mathematical property of the system, giving rise to the entire field of state estimation—Kalman filtering, particle filtering, hidden Markov models—as the principled response. In neuroscience, Helmholtz (1867) first formalized perception as an inference problem over hidden environmental states; Friston et al. (2017) developed this into the active inference framework that the AIG-ART architecture directly inherits. In pharmacokinetics, Jacquez and Perry (1990) demonstrated that drug distribution states are non-identifiable from plasma concentration curves alone, making structural identifiability analysis a prerequisite for any compartmental model. In population ecology, Ludwig et al. (1978) showed that fish population states cannot be recovered from catch data regardless of volume—a lesson learned through the collapse of fisheries managed entirely on observable outputs, in a failure mode structurally identical to tumor recurrence following apparent imaging response.

My identifiability analysis (Vaitheeswaran, 2026c) suggests that radiobiology may now be confronting a transition that several other quantitative disciplines faced earlier. It also reveals that observable treatment response may underdetermine the underlying tumor organization generating it. Similar patterns in fields such as control engineering, neuroscience, and systems biology eventually led to frameworks that treated hidden system state not as a nuisance variable, but as the central object of analysis. The recurring failures of mechanistic convergence across FLASH, SFRT, SBRT, and adaptive resistance suggest that radiobiology may be approaching a similar point.

Local Coherence Is Not Global Coherence

The old parable of the blind men and the elephant is usually told as a lesson about the limits of partial observation: each man touches one part of the animal—the trunk, the leg, the ear, the tail—and each declares the elephant to be a snake, a tree, a fan, a rope. The standard moral is that they are all wrong, because each generalises from a fragment.

But this is not quite the right reading. Each man's local report is exactly correct. The trunk really is rope-like. The leg really is column-like. The ear really is fan-like. There is no error of measurement, no failure of careful attention. Every individual description, taken at the scale at which it was made, is faithful to what is actually there. The men are not wrong locally. They are wrong only when their local descriptions are assembled into a global claim about what the animal is—and the gluing fails because the elephant is not the sum of its locally describable parts. It is an organism whose properties—how it moves, how it responds, how it behaves as a whole—depend on a structure that no individual touch can resolve.

This is the structural problem with mechanistic radiobiology. Each individual mechanism is locally correct. Oxygen depletion does happen. Bystander signalling does propagate.

Vascular damage does compromise tumour delivery. The molecular pathways that govern cellular response to radiation operate exactly as the literature describes. None of these claims is wrong locally. What is wrong is the assumption that gluing the local pictures together yields a global picture. The failures across FLASH, SFRT, and SBRT are not failures of mechanism. They are failures at exactly the scale where local mechanism stops governing and global organization begins. A description can be locally coherent at every point and still globally incoherent—and a system whose behaviour depends on its global organization cannot be predicted by accumulating local descriptions, however accurate each of them is.

The Resistance Connection

There is a specific place where this limitation becomes clinically consequential in a way that connects directly to the thread introduced in Chapter 1.

If the identifiability problem is genuine—if different internal configurations of the tumor can produce identical observable behavior—then it is impossible to predict, from baseline measurements alone, which configuration the tumor currently occupies. And if it is impossible to determine the current configuration, it is impossible to predict which configurations will emerge under the selective pressure of treatment.

This is the mechanistic account of why resistance is so hard to predict. Not because we lack biological knowledge—we have enormous biological knowledge. But because the internal state that determines which configurations are reachable under treatment pressure is not uniquely determined by the measurements we take. Two tumors that appear identical in every measured dimension may be in entirely different states—states that will lead them along entirely different trajectories under the same treatment.

The tumor is inferring its environment through the selection process. That inference operates on its internal state. And we cannot observe the internal state directly. This is not a failure of diligence. It is a structural feature of the problem.

Solving it requires not more mechanistic detail, but a different kind of description—one that explicitly represents the hidden internal state, tracks its evolution under perturbation, and provides principled methods for inferring it from the partial observations we can make. This is what the framework developed in the subsequent chapters attempts to provide.

What Is Required

The shift required is conceptual before it is technical. Instead of asking what mechanisms are present and what parameters they have, we need to ask: what is the organizational state of the system at this moment, how did it get there, and how will it evolve under intervention?

These questions require a representation of the system's state—its current configuration in a space defined by the constraints that govern its dynamics—and a framework for reasoning about how that state evolves over time and under external perturbation. This is the language of dynamical systems theory, of control theory, of statistical inference over hidden states. Not replacement of the mechanistic account—

extension of it. The mechanisms remain, but are now understood as components within an organizational framework rather than as the framework itself.

The tumor is not merely a collection of pathways. It is a system with state. And understanding that state—how it forms, how it changes, what it constrains—is the necessary next step.

The following chapters build that understanding from the ground up. We begin with what it means to say that a system has memory—not in any metaphorical sense, but in the precise dynamical sense that its present behavior carries forward the influence of its past.

CHAPTER

07

From Cells to Systems: Networks, Dynamics, and Emergence

The previous chapter closed with a question that the mechanistic program cannot answer on its own terms: what is the organizational state of the tumor, and how does it evolve? To answer it, we need a different way of thinking about what a tumor is.

The default picture is cellular. A tumor is a mass of cells—malignant cells with particular genetic mutations, surrounded by a supporting cast of immune cells, fibroblasts, and vasculature. Each cell has properties. Each cell responds to its environment. The tumor's behavior is, in this picture, the aggregate of its cellular constituents.

This picture describes what the tumor contains. It does not describe what the tumor is—which is something more than a collection of cells. It is a system. And the distinction between a collection and a system is not semantic. It is the difference between asking what the parts are and asking how they behave together.

What Makes Something a System

The word "system" is used loosely in biology, but it has a precise meaning in the scientific tradition we are drawing on here. A system is defined not primarily by its components but by the relationships between them—the interactions that connect components, the feedback loops that link cause and effect across time, and the organizational properties that emerge from these interactions and cannot be attributed to any single component (Bertalanffy, 1968; Kitano, 2002).

The shift from components to systems is not merely a change in scale. It is a change in the kinds of questions that become answerable. When you ask about components, you ask: what is this made of? What are its properties? When you ask about systems, you ask: how is this organized? How does it change? What does it do that its parts cannot do alone?

Both sets of questions matter. But for predicting tumor behavior under treatment—particularly the behavior that current models fail to capture—the systems questions are the ones that need to be asked.

The Tumor as a Network

Within a tumor, interactions are pervasive and multidirectional. Cancer cells signal to each other through paracrine and autocrine pathways, coordinating behavior across populations. They signal to stromal cells—fibroblasts, endothelial cells, immune cells—and receive signals back, creating a dense web of intercellular communication (Hanahan and Weinberg, 2011; Junttila and de Sauvage, 2013). Vascular architecture determines which regions receive oxygen and nutrients, creating spatial gradients that organize the tumor's ecology. The extracellular matrix provides mechanical cues that influence cell migration, proliferation, and differentiation (Jain, 1987).

These interactions form a network—a literal network of causal relationships, where the state of any node influences the states of others, and where the network's global properties cannot be read off from its individual nodes (Barabási and Oltvai, 2004). The tumor is, in this precise sense, a networked dynamical system—one that inherits the rich organizational structure of gene regulatory networks, signaling networks, and metabolic networks (Alon, 2007), and adds to it the spatial and temporal organization produced by tumor growth, treatment, and adaptation.

Dynamics: The Behavior of Networks Over Time

A network's structure determines what kinds of dynamics are possible. But structure alone does not determine what actually happens—dynamics depend on initial conditions, on the strength of interactions, and on how the network responds to perturbations.

Biological networks are rich in two kinds of feedback that are particularly important for understanding tumor behavior. Positive feedback loops amplify perturbations—small changes propagate and grow, enabling rapid transitions between states. Negative feedback loops stabilize behavior—deviations from a reference state are corrected, maintaining robustness. When these two types of feedback are combined and coupled, the resulting dynamics can be remarkably complex: bistability, where the system maintains two distinct stable states and can switch between them; oscillations, where the system cycles repeatedly through a sequence of states; and sensitivity to initial conditions, where small differences in starting configuration lead to large differences in long-term behavior (Tyson and Novak, 2010; Alon, 2007).

These are not exotic phenomena. They are generic properties of biological regulatory networks. The lac operon switches between induced and uninduced states. The cell cycle oscillates between growth and division phases. Developmental decisions—the commitment of a stem cell to a particular lineage—are governed by bistable switches that, once crossed, are maintained through positive feedback (Ferrell, 2002). These examples are canonical in cell biology. Their relevance to tumor behavior is direct.

A tumor that contains bistable regulatory circuits can exist in multiple distinct phenotypic states—not as a continuum of responses, but as discrete configurations with qualitatively different properties. Resistance, on this view, is not a gradual drift along a continuous spectrum. It is a transition between states—from a sensitive configuration to a resistant one. The transition has a threshold. Once crossed, it is maintained by positive feedback. This is exactly the kind of behavior that continuous dose-response models cannot represent, and exactly the kind of behavior that SBRT appears to trigger.

Emergence: When the Whole Exceeds Its Parts

The most important concept for understanding what systems offer that component-level descriptions cannot is emergence. Emergent properties are properties of the system as a whole that cannot be attributed to or predicted from the properties of the individual components. They arise from interactions—from the way components relate to and constrain each other—not from the components themselves.

Emergence is not mystical. It is a mathematical consequence of the fact that interacting components collectively explore a state space that no single component occupies alone. Water is wet because of how H_2O molecules interact with each other; no individual molecule has the property of wetness. A flock of starlings displays coordinated movement that no individual bird plans; the coordination emerges from local interaction rules followed by each bird (Camazine et al., 2001).

In tumors, several clinically important properties are emergent in this sense. Coordinated resistance—the simultaneous shift of a cell population toward therapy-resistant phenotypes—is not simply the sum of individual cells becoming resistant. It involves communication between cells, reorganization of the tumor microenvironment, and collective dynamics that depend on the network's global state (Marusyk et al., 2012). The capacity for long-range spatial effects—the ability of perturbations to propagate across the tumor in ways that affect distant, unirradiated regions—is an emergent property of the network's connectivity, not a property of any individual cell or signaling molecule. The apparent "decision" of a tumor to shift from one growth pattern to another is an emergent consequence of the network crossing a threshold in state space.

These emergent properties are causally real. They shape clinical outcomes. And they are precisely what gets lost when tumors are analyzed as collections of independent components.

Two experimental results make this concrete in ways that directly challenge the genomic reductionist account of tumor behavior. Gupta et al. (2011) demonstrated that distinct phenotypic states in breast cancer cell lines—basal, luminal, and stem-like—interconvert stochastically, and that a population purified to a single phenotypic state spontaneously regenerates the full heterogeneous mixture within days. The equilibrium proportions are determined not by the genome but by the organizational dynamics of the population. This is direct experimental proof that the hidden state is not genomic—that it exists at the population organizational level and evolves independently of any genomic change. Marusyk et al. (2014) extended this further, demonstrating that minority subpopulations within tumors can drive the collective behavior of the majority through paracrine signaling—a small number of cells in a particular organizational state reshaping what the entire tumor does in ways entirely invisible to measurements of the majority population's genomic composition. Together these results establish experimentally what the systems perspective demands theoretically: that collective tumor behavior is an emergent organizational property, not a sum of individual cellular properties, and that the hidden state governing that behavior is neither genomic nor recoverable from any measurement of individual components.

Variability as Organizational Information

This systems perspective reframes clinical variability in a way that has important practical consequences.

In the standard view, variability in treatment response across patients is noise—the unpredictable spread of biological characteristics across a population. It is managed statistically, by averaging over populations and identifying central tendencies. It is reduced, in principle, by better characterization of individual patients.

In the systems view, variability is not noise. It is information. Different patients differ not merely in their measured molecular characteristics but in the organizational state of their tumor systems—the configuration of the network at the time of treatment, the history of prior exposures that shaped that configuration, and the position in state space from which treatment is initiating the dynamical trajectory. Two tumors that appear identical in measured molecular characteristics can be in different organizational states, and those states will determine their trajectories under treatment.

This means that variability cannot be eliminated by measuring more molecular variables, because the variables that determine variability are not molecular properties of individual components but organizational properties of the system as a whole. The variability is real and irreducible at the component level. It becomes tractable only when described at the level of the system's state.

Bioelectric Networks as Organizational Infrastructure

There is one specific kind of network that deserves particular attention here, because it operates at a level of organization that conventional molecular analysis tends to miss and that has direct relevance to both tumor behavior and treatment response.

Every cell in the body maintains a resting membrane potential—a voltage difference between its interior and exterior, maintained by the activity of ion channels and pumps. What Levin and colleagues have demonstrated is that patterns of membrane potential across a tissue—bioelectric fields—encode organizational information that governs cell behavior at the collective level: directing growth, maintaining tissue boundaries, and providing long-range coordination that biochemical signaling alone cannot achieve (Levin, 2021; Levin et al., 2021). Cancer involves a disruption of this bioelectric organization—tumor cells show characteristic depolarization that is not merely a consequence of malignant transformation but a causal contributor to it (Levin, 2021; Chernet and Levin, 2014).

The tumor is therefore organized at multiple levels simultaneously—genetic, epigenetic, signaling network, bioelectric field—and understanding its behavior requires engaging with all of these levels and the relationships between them. Chapter 10 develops the bioelectric evidence in full. What matters here is the structural point: bioelectric networks are one concrete instantiation of the kind of organizational infrastructure that makes tumours behave as systems rather than collections.

From System to State

The systems perspective developed in this chapter leads naturally to a crucial concept that will become central to everything that follows. If the tumor is a networked dynamical system—if its behavior depends on how its components interact, on the feedback loops connecting them, on the emergent properties arising from their collective dynamics—then at any given moment, the tumor occupies a specific position in the space of possible configurations. That position—the tumor's current configuration across all its relevant dimensions—determines how it will respond to any given intervention.

This position is what we mean by the system's state. Not a list of measured variables, but the full organizational configuration of the system at a given moment, including all the history-dependent, feedback-shaped, emergent properties that the variables we measure are only partial projections of.

A system with memory carries its past forward in its state. The current state reflects what the system has experienced, and constrains what it can become. And this is where the resistance thread from Chapter 1 gains its systems-level grounding. Resistance is not cells becoming resistant. It is the system transitioning to a state in which resistant configurations are stable and sensitive configurations are not. That transition is a property of the system's dynamics—its feedback structure, its bistability, its sensitivity to perturbation. It cannot be understood at the level of individual cells or individual mechanisms. It requires the language of state and dynamics.

The next chapter asks: what exactly does it mean for a system to carry its past forward? What is the nature of biological memory, understood not as a neural phenomenon but as a property of any networked dynamical system capable of history-dependent behavior?

CHAPTER

08

Memory and History Dependence

The previous chapter established that tumors are networked dynamical systems—organized entities whose collective behavior emerges from interactions between components across multiple levels simultaneously. One consequence of this follows with mathematical necessity: such systems carry their past forward into their present behavior.

This is what we mean by memory. Not memory in the neural sense—not storage and retrieval of discrete information by a specialized structure. Memory in the dynamical sense: the influence of prior states on current behavior, encoded not in any single location but distributed across the system's current configuration. A system with memory is one whose response to an identical input depends on the history of inputs that preceded it. And as the previous chapters documented across three different experimental domains, this is precisely what tumors appear to be.

The question this chapter addresses is: what is the biological basis of this memory? Is it a vague metaphor, or is there concrete experimental evidence that biological systems—even simple ones, far simpler than tumors—genuinely exhibit this property?

The evidence, as it turns out, is both recent and striking.

Memory Beyond the Brain

For most of scientific history, memory was considered a property of nervous systems. Neurons are specialized precisely for this function—they form connections, strengthen them through use, and thereby encode the history of past activity in a form that shapes future responses. The brain's capacity for memory is the result of billions of years of evolution producing dedicated cellular machinery.

What recent work has demonstrated is that memory, understood as history-dependent behavior modification, is not confined to neurons. It is a property of biological networks far more generally—arising not from specialized memory machinery but from the fundamental dynamics of any system capable of nonlinear feedback.

The most striking demonstration of this principle comes from single cells. In a series of experiments that have attracted considerable attention, researchers showed that Stentor coeruleus—a single-celled organism, a protozoan without a nervous system of any kind—can form associative relationships between stimuli (Doan et al., 2026). Exposed to paired presentations of two stimuli over time, the organism modifies its behavior in ways that anticipate the second stimulus upon presentation of the first alone. This is associative conditioning—the same fundamental form of learning described by Pavlov in dogs—occurring in a cell that has no neurons, no synapses, and no brain.

The implication is significant. Associative memory is not a neural phenomenon. It is a dynamical phenomenon—a consequence of how certain kinds of networks process information over time. The hardware of neurons is one way to implement this capability. It is not the only way.

Gene Regulatory Networks as Learning Systems

At the molecular level, Pigozzi, Goldstein, and Levin demonstrated something equally remarkable (Pigozzi et al., 2025). Gene regulatory networks—the circuits of transcription factors and signaling molecules that govern gene expression—can be trained using paradigms directly analogous to Pavlovian conditioning. When exposed to paired stimuli in a defined temporal sequence, the network modifies its future responses in ways that reflect the learned association. The genetic sequence is unchanged. The connectivity of the network is unchanged. What changes is the dynamic state of the network—the configuration of expression levels and regulatory activities that the network has been brought to through the training experience.

This is memory as state, not memory as storage. The network does not add a dedicated memory module. It changes itself—its dynamic configuration—in a way that encodes the prior experience and makes it accessible to future responses. Remove the experience and the memory fades. Reapply it and the memory returns, often more readily than the first time. The system learns.

A further finding from this work deserves emphasis because it changes how we think about what learning does to a system. Associative training in gene regulatory networks does not merely change response patterns. It increases what Pigozzi and colleagues call causal emergence—a measure of how much the system's behavior is governed by its collective state rather than by the independent dynamics of its individual components (Pigozzi et al., 2025). In plain terms: before training, the network behaves more like a collection of semi-independent parts. After training, it behaves more like a unified whole. The parts become more strongly coupled to each other. The system becomes more integrated.

This is a deep result. Memory, in biological networks, does not just record the past. It reorganizes the system—strengthening the coupling between components, increasing the degree to which the system acts as a coherent entity rather than a collection of parts. Learning creates integration. And integration, as we saw in Chapter 7, is precisely what gives systems their emergent properties.

The Experimental Ground Has Shifted

Let me pause here, because what these results mean for this book specifically deserves to be stated plainly.

The organizational picture of cancer—that tumors behave as systems with memory, that they integrate experience, that their hidden state governs their response—has been argued compellingly before. Davies and Lineweaver (2011) built the evolutionary case. Levin (2021) built the bioelectric case. Mukherjee (2022) built the clinical-biological case. Each arrived at essentially the same conclusion by a different route. But each was arguing from inference: from theoretical necessity, from developmental biology in model organisms, from the accumulated weight of experimental observation pointing in a consistent direction. None had direct experimental demonstration that a non-neural biological network learns an association, integrates that learning as a measurable change in organizational structure, and can have that learning selectively reversed.

Pigozzi et al. (2025) and Doan et al. (2026) provide exactly that. The experimental ground has shifted. What was previously a conclusion forced by inference is now a conclusion supported by direct demonstration. And this shift has a specific consequence for how we should think about tumor response to radiotherapy.

If biological networks learn—and they demonstrably do—then a tumor under repeated radiation exposure is not merely adapting stochastically. It is integrating the information content of the treatment being applied and reorganizing its internal configuration accordingly. Pigozzi et al. showed that this reorganization is not merely behavioral but structural: learning increases causal emergence, meaning the network's parts become more strongly coupled as a consequence of the learning process. Applied to the tumor, this prediction has a precise clinical signature. Resistance—the tumor's learned response to a treatment policy—should not only change the tumor's behavior. It should change its organizational structure. It should increase the degree to which the tumor's regions are coupled, coordinated, and mutually predictive. A rising organizational integration, visible in the tumor's spatial dynamics before it is visible in any conventional imaging metric, is the expected fingerprint of a system that has learned its treatment rather than merely survived it.

The clinical measurement framework capable of detecting exactly this signature—and what it implies for treatment decisions—is developed in Chapter 12.

Memory Can Be Selectively Erased

A further property of this kind of memory is that it is not permanent. Pigozzi and colleagues also demonstrated that memories encoded in gene regulatory networks can be selectively erased through targeted interventions—returning the network to a less conditioned state—without disrupting the network's overall structure or its capacity to learn again (Pigozzi et al., 2025). The memory is not hard-wired. It is a dynamic property of the system's current state, not of its fixed architecture.

If resistance is a state—if a tumor has learned to resist a particular treatment through a dynamic encoding of prior exposure—then strategies that perturb the state, rather than simply escalating the same intervention, may be able to reset or redirect that learned configuration. The tumor's memory can potentially be disrupted. We will return to this in Part IV.

Memory Is Distributed, Not Localized

One of the counterintuitive properties of network memory is its distribution. In systems like gene regulatory networks, no individual component contains the memory. Different parts of the network experience different aspects of the training stimulus. No single node has access to the full history. Yet the memory emerges from the network as a whole—from the pattern of interactions and state variables distributed across all the components simultaneously (Pigozzi et al., 2025).

This distributed nature has an important consequence for measurement. If memory is distributed across the system's state, it cannot be detected by measuring any individual component. Measuring one gene's expression level, one signaling molecule's concentration, one biomarker's value—none of these captures the organizational state in which the memory is encoded. The measurement has to be of the system's collective behavior, or the memory remains invisible.

This is precisely the problem we encountered in Chapter 6 with the identifiability issue. The internal state that governs behavior—including the history-dependent, memory-like configuration of the system—is not accessible from measurements of individual components. It requires inference from the system's collective dynamics, which is exactly what the framework developed in subsequent chapters provides.

Memory in Tissue: The Bioelectric Layer

The memory demonstrated in gene regulatory networks and single cells operates at the molecular and cellular scale. Whether analogous memory properties exist at the tissue scale is answered directly by Levin and colleagues' experimental work on bioelectric patterns—distributed maps of membrane potential across cell populations that organize tissue behavior through long-range electrical signaling (Levin, 2021; Levin et al., 2021). In planaria, transient disruption of the bioelectric state during regeneration produces two-headed worms that continue regenerating two-headed animals indefinitely through subsequent cuttings—long after the pharmacological perturbation has cleared completely (Levin, 2014). The genome is unchanged. The memory is stored in the bioelectric organizational state and persists biophysically. Chapter 10 develops this evidence in full. What matters here is the principle: tissue-level memory encoded in dynamic bioelectric state, not in DNA, is a demonstrated biological reality—and precisely the kind of distributed, state-encoded memory the systems perspective predicts.

The Persistence of Memory Under Treatment

Biological memory of this kind persists well beyond the training period—gene regulatory network memory continues after training stimuli are removed (Pigozzi et al., 2025), and bioelectric memory in planaria persists through unlimited regeneration cycles. In bistable systems, this is expected: the stability of the state itself maintains the memory without continuous active effort.

Assembly Theory offers a complementary and more fundamental account of this durability. Defined by Cronin, Walker and colleagues, the molecular assembly index measures the minimum number of steps required to construct an object from its elementary building blocks—and demonstrates that objects requiring many such steps could not have arisen without a selection process (Marshall et al., 2021; Sharma et al., 2023). Applied to the tumour's organisational state: each layer of adaptive response—epigenetic, bioelectric, clonal—adds assembly steps whose irreversibility is encoded in the current configuration. Reaching a qualitatively different organisational state of comparable complexity requires comparably many steps. The memory is durable not only because feedback maintains it, but because the construction that produced it was irreversible.

Assembly Theory provides a complementary perspective on why such internal states, once formed, persist. Systems whose structure arises through sequences of constrained, non-random assembly steps necessarily encode aspects of that history in their present configuration. In this sense, the system's current state is not independent of its past, but a physical record of it. While not specific to tumor biology, this framework supports the view that history-dependent internal states can be stably realized in material systems, rather than being transient or purely conceptual.

In the clinical context, this means that the history a tumor has accumulated during treatment is not erased between fractions.

Each treatment fraction encounters a tumor that has been modified by all prior fractions. The system is not reset. It remembers. This is why sequence matters, as the temporal problem in Chapter 2 demonstrated. And it is why radiotherapy that ignores the history-dependent state of the tumor is, in a precise sense, incomplete—it is acting on a system without accounting for where that system is in its state space, and where it has been

Memory Defines the System

There is a philosophical point here that is worth making explicitly, because it changes how we think about what kind of thing a tumor is.

A memoryless system or a Markovian system is fully described by its current state. Its past is irrelevant—wash it out, reset the initial conditions, and the system behaves as though nothing preceded the current moment. Many physical systems approximate this ideal, and it is the assumption that underlies much of classical physics and conventional radiobiology.

A system with memory (non-Markovian) is not fully described by its current measurable state. Its past is embedded in its present in ways that shape its future behavior but are not directly visible in any single snapshot. To understand such a system, you must understand its trajectory—the path it has taken through state space, not just where it is now.

Tumors are systems with memory. Their response to any intervention depends on what they have already experienced. The history of prior treatment, of growth, of hypoxia and reoxygenation, of immune pressure—all of this is encoded in the system's current organizational state, shaping which transitions are accessible, which configurations are stable, and which responses are available.

This is not simply a statement about biological complexity. It is a statement about the kind of mathematical object a tumor is—and therefore about the kind of framework needed to reason about it. A system with memory requires a representation of its state, a model of how that state evolves, and a method for inferring the state from incomplete observations. These are not features of the conventional radiobiological toolkit. They are features of the framework built in the chapters that follow.

If memory is embedded in the system's organizational state, then the next question is how to define and represent that state formally. What captures the system at a given moment in a way that reflects its history and determines its future?

That is the question Chapter 9 addresses.

CHAPTER

09

The Informational State and Top-Down Causation

From Memory to Encoding

Memory, as established in Chapter 8, cannot exist without physical instantiation. If past states influence present behavior—if the system responds differently to the same input depending on what preceded it—then the influence of those past states must leave a trace in the system's current condition. That trace is not a record, stored somewhere and retrieved on demand. It is a constraint: the current organizational configuration of the system, shaped by all prior states, which determines what future states are accessible and which are not.

This is the precise relationship between memory and information. Information, in the sense most relevant here, is not messages or symbols. It is what constrains the possible states a system can occupy. A system without memory can, in principle, evolve toward any configuration accessible from its current position. A system with memory cannot—its past has restricted the space of accessible futures. Those restrictions are information, physically instantiated in the system's current organizational state (Shannon, 1948; Jaynes, 1957).

The implication follows with logical necessity: memory implies encoding, and encoding implies a structured internal state. If past states influence present behavior, that influence must be physically present within the system as a constraint on its future evolution. Not as a label or a record—as structure. As organization. As the current configuration that prior experience has shaped into something that is not neutral with respect to what can happen next.

This structured internal state is what we define as the informational state.

What kind of internal state could produce the pattern of failures documented in Part I? The alternatives can be enumerated precisely. A purely stochastic description is insufficient: while stochastic systems can generate variability, they do not, by themselves, account for the systematic, threshold-like, and directional patterns observed in FLASH, SFRT, and SBRT.

A purely genomic state is likewise incomplete. Experimental work (Gupta, 2011; Marusyk, 2014; Flavahan, 2017) demonstrates that clinically relevant tumor states can transition without corresponding genomic change, indicating that genetic variation alone cannot account for the observed dynamics.

A purely metabolic state captures important aspects of local radiosensitivity, but does not, in isolation, explain the coordinated spatial coupling or the history-dependent, directional adaptation seen across treatments.

A purely microenvironmental description is clearly relevant, but is better understood as part of the substrate in which the state is realized, rather than a complete characterization of the state itself.

Taken together, these considerations indicate that no single class of variables—stochastic, genomic, metabolic, or microenvironmental—provides a sufficient description on its own. Each captures an aspect of the system, but none accounts for the full pattern of behavior observed. What remains, therefore, is a state that integrates these components into an organized, history-dependent, and causally active configuration. This conclusion follows directly from the structure of the observed phenomena, which cannot be accounted for by models lacking such a state.

Independent work in the physics of living systems has argued that biological organization is maintained through informational constraints that act on physical processes (Davies, 2019). While not derived in the context of radiotherapy, these results support the interpretation that the required internal state is not merely a collection of physical variables, but an organized, information-bearing configuration that guides system behavior. We therefore interpret the required internal state as an informational state: an organized, history-dependent configuration that encodes constraints on system evolution and governs its response to perturbation.

The informational state is therefore not an external assumption imposed on the data, but a consistent interpretation of both the empirical failures of classical models and broader theoretical perspectives on living systems.

Defining the Informational State

We define the informational state of the tumor—denoted s_t—as the set of constraints, at time t, that determine the system's possible transitions.

The informational state is not a list of measured variables. It is the full organizational configuration of the system—the pattern of gene regulatory activity, epigenetic modifications, signaling network states, spatial distribution of phenotypic configurations, and tissue-level bioelectric organization—all considered simultaneously, as they constrain each other and collectively determine what the system can and cannot do next. It is not what we can see. It is what is there, of which what we see is only a partial and imperfect projection.

Three properties follow from this definition and will be carried forward through the rest of the book.

The informational state is history-dependent. s_t reflects where the system has been. The current configuration was shaped by prior treatment, prior adaptive responses, prior selective pressure. Two tumors with identical measured profiles at time t may have arrived at that configuration via entirely different histories, placing them in different informational states that will generate different trajectories under the same subsequent treatment.

The informational state is distributed. s_t is not localized in any single component or any single measurement dimension. Like the memory demonstrated in gene regulatory networks and bioelectric tissue fields in Chapter 8, the informational state is a property of the whole system, encoded across all its components and the relationships between them simultaneously.

The informational state is only partially observable. What clinical measurement provides—imaging signals, molecular markers, treatment responses—are projections of s_t onto the dimensions that current instruments can access. These projections carry information about the state, but as the identifiability problem established in Chapter 6, they do not uniquely determine it. Different underlying states can produce identical projections. The state is real. The measurement is incomplete.

And critically—the one property that this chapter must establish carefully—the informational state is causally active. It does not merely describe the system. It governs it.

The Argument for Causal Power

This is the claim that requires the most care, because it runs against the default framework of molecular biology and conventional radiobiology. In those frameworks, causation flows upward: molecular events produce cellular behaviors, cellular behaviors produce tissue properties, tissue properties produce clinical outcomes. This is bottom-up causation, and it has been enormously productive. The question is whether it is sufficient.

Consider a simple observation that the bottom-up framework struggles to explain. The same molecular components—the same oncogene, the same cell type, the same signaling molecules—can produce radically different behaviors depending on their organizational context. An oncogenic mutation that drives aggressive proliferation in one tissue organization can be completely suppressed in a different organizational context without any change in the molecular machinery. The oncogene is present and active at the molecular level. The organizational state of the tissue—something about how cells are connected, what signals they are receiving from their collective configuration, what bioelectric field they are embedded in—overrides it.

This has been demonstrated experimentally, and the evidence is presented in full detail in Chapter 10. Here, the logical point is sufficient: if the same molecular components produce different outcomes in different organizational contexts, then the organizational context is doing causal work. It is determining the outcome. Something at the level of the whole is governing what happens at the level of the parts. This is top-down causation—not as a philosophical preference but as an empirical observation that the molecular framework cannot accommodate without invoking organizational state (Ellis, 2012; Campbell, 1974; Davies, 2019).

Constraints as the Form of Causation

The most precise way to understand how the informational state exerts its causal influence is through the concept of constraints. The state does not push the system's components in any particular direction. It shapes the space within which they move—defining which transitions are accessible and which are not, which trajectories are possible and which are blocked.

A small example. At home, my niece Vedha moves through the house without constraint—talking loudly, interrupting freely, ignoring most attempts at structure. In a temple, she does something different. She lowers her voice, stays close, watches what others are doing before she acts—the place carries rules she can sense but no one has stated. The same child. A different setting.

Seen this way, her behaviour is less a set of choices than a trajectory shaped by the environment. Like a ball rolling across a surface, she moves differently depending on the contours she is in. On one surface, the motion is free and unconstrained. On another, it is guided, limited, redirected. The parts have not changed. The landscape has.

The informational state operates in precisely this way. Local molecular processes—the binding and unbinding of transcription factors, the firing of signaling cascades, the opening and closing of ion channels—occur according to the laws of biochemistry and biophysics. But they occur within a landscape defined by the informational state: a landscape that makes some outcomes probable, others improbable, and others effectively inaccessible. The local processes are bottom-up. The landscape is determined top-down by the organizational state. Ellis and Davies have formalized this insight: higher-level organizational structure sets boundary conditions within which lower-level processes operate, and information in living systems acts as a causal determinant of physical processes rather than merely a description of them (Ellis, 2012; Davies, 2012; Davies, 2019).

Why This Matters for Radiobiology

If the informational state is causally active—if it constrains which tumor behaviors are accessible and which are not—then the response to any given treatment is not determined solely by the physical dose delivered and the molecular properties of the cells receiving it. It is determined by the combination of that dose and the organizational state of the system at the time of delivery. Two identical doses, delivered to tumors in different informational states, will initiate different trajectories. Two tumors that appear molecularly identical, that show the same imaging features, that have received the same treatment history, can nevertheless be in different informational states—states that lead them to respond differently to the same next fraction.

This is not variability to be reduced by better measurement of molecular variables. It is variability that reflects genuine organizational differences that no molecular measurement can fully capture. The identifiability problem is not a gap that more data will close. It is a structural feature of the relationship between the informational state and its observable projections.

There is also a resistance implication that connects directly to the thread established in Chapter 1. If the tumor's informational state constrains what transitions are accessible, then the state shapes which resistant configurations can be reached under treatment pressure. Resistance is not cells randomly acquiring mutations that happen to confer survival advantage. It is the system's organizational state—shaped by the history of prior treatment—making certain configurations more accessible than others. The treatment is providing information to the system. The system is integrating that information into its state. And the evolved state increasingly reflects what the system has been taught by the treatment being applied. This is resistance as inference—now formalised here in the language of the informational state—and it operates at the level of organizational state, not at the level of individual cellular mechanisms.

The game-theoretic implication follows: a treatment policy that is predictable enough for the tumor's evolutionary dynamics to learn will eventually be overcome by the state's adaptation to it. A policy that changes faster than the state can adapt maintains the advantage. AIG-ART, as developed in Part IV, is designed precisely around this insight.

What the State Is and What It Is Not

Two clarifications are necessary before we proceed further.

First, the informational state is not a new variable to be added to existing models. It is a different level of description—one that represents the organizational configuration of the system rather than the values of individual molecular parameters. Mechanistic models describe what the components are and what they do individually. The informational state describes how they are organized collectively and what that organization permits and prohibits. These descriptions are complementary but not equivalent. The organizational level captures something the molecular level cannot: the causal role of the whole in governing its parts.

Second, saying the state is only partially observable is not the same as saying it is unknowable. It can be inferred—partially, probabilistically, with uncertainty that decreases as more observations accumulate. The belief state $b_t(s) = p(s_t = s \mid o_1{:}t, a_1{:}t_{-1})$ is the formal representation of this inference: a probability distribution over possible states, updated as new observations arrive. The full machinery of this inference—how it is computed, how it guides action selection, how it connects to the AIG-ART treatment architecture—is developed in Chapter 13 and formalized in Appendix A.

The Status of the Framework: Three Readings

The argument of this chapter—that the informational state s_t is real, causally active, and not reducible to any set of molecular measurements—can be read in three distinct ways. These readings do not concern whether the informational state exists—that question is settled by the elimination of alternatives and by Davies's physical argument inherited above. They concern how strongly to read its ontological status. Physics has faced this before. Quantum mechanics was used to build transistors and lasers long before there was agreement on what the wavefunction actually is. Different interpretations coexisted—instrumental, realist, and agnostic—while the theory itself was tested and applied. The same structure appears here: the following readings differ in how seriously they take the ontology, not in whether the framework can be used.

The pragmatic reading. The organizational level of description is the useful one, regardless of whether it is the fundamental one—just as thermodynamics remains indispensable in engineering despite being derivable in principle from statistical mechanics. On this reading, s_t is a scaffold defined at the level where the relevant dynamics are tractable. Readers who believe the organizational level is ultimately eliminable lose nothing of the clinical argument: the four-component state vector, the belief state $b_t(s)$, the POMDP architecture, the AIG-ART treatment policy—all are worth pursuing whether or not the organizational level is ontologically autonomous.

The stronger reading, which this book defends. The organizational level is not merely convenient but causally autonomous—the constraints the informational state imposes on component behavior are real in a sense that no future supercomputer would dissolve. In macroeconomics, Lucas demonstrated that ignoring organizational states of agents produces systematic, predictable policy failures (Lucas, 1976). In ecology, the collapse of cod fisheries showed that population states are not recoverable from aggregate outputs—a failure mode structurally identical to tumour recurrence following apparent imaging response (Ludwig et al., 1978). In each case, the emergent organizational description became the primary object of the science. The identifiability result here is not a practical limitation. It is structural. The organizational level is where the relevant causal structure lives.

The honest reading: a disciplined what-if. The biological evidence that non-neural systems encode history as organizational state is direct and demonstrated. Pigozzi et al. (2025) showed that gene regulatory networks learn associations in the precise Pavlovian sense. Doan et al. (2026) demonstrated the same in a single cell with no nervous system. The planarian experiments of Levin and colleagues—fully detailed in Chapter 10—show that bioelectric organizational state can be permanently rewritten by a transient physiological perturbation. These experiments establish that the kind of thing this book is proposing exists in biology. What remains inferential is the specific claim that tumours possess such a state in ways that govern their response to radiotherapy. The ghost has been located by triangulation. It has not been seen. The framework can therefore be read as a disciplined what-if—one whose predictions are specific enough to be wrong, and whose wrongness, if demonstrated, would itself be scientifically informative. Appendix D registers those predictions. That register is the framework's commitment to accountability.

What all three readings share: the clinical and scientific argument of this book stands on all three. The pragmatic reading is sufficient for everything that follows. The disciplined what-if is the posture the framework actually occupies as a body of work—proposing, not proving. The stronger reading is one philosophical interpretation available to readers who find it compelling. The framework requires only that the what-if be taken seriously enough to test. The following chapter provides the most compelling current reason to do so.

Three Questions That Follow

The theoretical argument of this chapter leads naturally to three empirical questions that the framework alone cannot answer.

First: what is the informational state physically made of—what are the physical substrates in real biological tissue that carry this organizational information and make it causally active?

Second: can the informational state be observed, even partially—are there clinically accessible measurements that give reliable partial views beyond the scalar summaries the identifiability problem renders blind to organizational structure?

Third: can the informational state be deliberately manipulated—is there evidence that biological organizational states can be shifted through physiological interventions that do not require changing the genetic sequence?

The answer to all three questions is yes—and the evidence is concrete, reproducible, and comes from some of the most striking experiments in modern developmental biology. That evidence is the subject of Chapter 10.

CHAPTER

10

The Biology of Top-Down Causation: Target Morphology and the Bioelectric Basis of the Informational State

The preceding chapter established the theoretical architecture of the informational state and ended with three specific questions: what the state is physically made of, whether it can be observed even partially, and whether it can be deliberately manipulated. This chapter answers all three—through biological evidence that is concrete, reproducible, and forces a reconception of what cancer is at its organizational core.

One clarification of logical structure is necessary before the experimental evidence is presented. Davies (2019) argues, on physical grounds, that living systems exhibiting goal-directed organizational maintenance are best understood as operating through causally active informational states. This perspective was adopted in Chapter 9 and is not re-derived here. What this chapter addresses is the subsequent and separable question: what is that state physically made of in biological tissue?

Levin's experimental work in planaria, *Xenopus*, and related model organisms provides the strongest available answer. It demonstrates that bioelectric field patterns—tissue-wide distributions of membrane potential maintained through gap junctional coupling—function as a memory mechanism encoding organisational information, alterable through physiological means and persistent without genomic change. This framework proposes that the same substrate, operating in clinical tumours under radiotherapy, is the biological basis of the informational state s_t. That proposal is an extension of Levin's findings, not an independent result of his experimental programme.

The Puzzle of Coordinated Tissue Behavior

Before examining the experiments, it is worth stating the puzzle they address, because the puzzle itself clarifies what the informational state must do.

When tissue regenerates after injury—or when an embryo develops from a single fertilized cell into a complex organism with precisely organized structures—billions of cells must coordinate their behavior toward a collective outcome. Each cell implements molecular programs. Each cell responds to local signals. But the final form is global, not local. A planarian flatworm, cut in half, regenerates not just the cells it lost but the correct proportions, the correct structures, the correct spatial organization of an entire animal. The cells at the wound site do not know in advance what structures are missing. They must somehow assess the current state of the fragment, compare it with a representation of the target configuration, and organize their behavior to close the gap.

No molecule provides this global information. Morphogen gradients are local—they tell a cell about its immediate neighborhood. Gene expression programs are intrinsic—they specify what molecular processes a cell can carry out. Neither, by itself, can account for the tissue-level coordination required to regenerate a complex structure from an arbitrary fragment, beginning from cells that were neighbors before the cut and therefore cannot be distinguished by local position alone.

Something else is providing the global organizational signal. Something that spans the entire tissue, that encodes the target the tissue is trying to achieve, and that coordinates the behavior of individual cells toward that target from above—constraining what they do individually in service of what the whole must become.

Levin and colleagues have proposed, and extensively demonstrated, that this global organizational signal is bioelectric in nature: a tissue-wide pattern of resting membrane potentials, maintained through the electrical coupling of cells via gap junctions, that encodes what they call the target morphology—the anatomical setpoint toward which the tissue's collective dynamics are organized (Pezzulo and Levin, 2016; Levin, 2021).

The Planarian Experiments

The experimental demonstration of this concept is most complete and most striking in planarian flatworms—small freshwater organisms with extraordinary regenerative capacity. When a planarian is cut into many pieces, each fragment regenerates into a complete, correctly proportioned worm. The cells in any fragment can give rise to any part of the body. The regenerating fragment "knows" what structures are missing and builds them—correctly, reliably, and with the right proportions relative to the remaining tissue.

The key question is: where is this knowledge stored? What encodes the target morphology—the specification of what a complete planarian should look like—and how is it communicated to the cells carrying out the regeneration?

The answer emerged from a deceptively simple intervention. When gap junctions—the electrical synapses that connect adjacent cells and allow membrane potentials to propagate across tissue—are transiently blocked during regeneration, the fragment does not regenerate normally. Instead of one head at the anterior wound and one tail at the posterior wound, it grows a head at both ends. A two-headed worm (Oviedo et al., 2010; Beane et al., 2011).

This result alone, while striking, might be interpreted as simply a disruption of the mechanism that distinguishes anterior from posterior. What makes it profound is what happens next. The gap junction blocker is washed out completely. Normal gap junctional connectivity is restored. The worm is then cut again—and it grows two heads again, without any further intervention. It is cut again. Two heads again. This continues indefinitely, through multiple rounds of regeneration, long after any trace of the pharmacological perturbation has dissipated from the tissue (Durant et al., 2017).

The genome is unchanged. The molecular machinery of individual cells is unchanged. The perturbation that caused the change is gone. And yet the tissue continues to build two-headed animals—because the bioelectric circuit that encodes the target morphology has been permanently rewritten. A brief, purely physiological disruption to the tissue's electrical connectivity has altered the organizational memory that governs what shape the tissue regenerates toward, and that altered memory maintains itself through the tissue's own dynamics, indefinitely.

This is tissue-level memory—physically instantiated in the bioelectric state of the tissue, not in the genetic sequence of its cells. It was created by a physiological perturbation. It persists without continuous maintenance. It can be read out through subsequent regeneration events. And it is, in precisely the sense established in Chapter 9, top-down causation: the organizational state of the tissue determining what individual cells do, overriding the bottom-up signals that would otherwise direct normal anterior-posterior patterning.

What Target Morphology Is

Target morphology, in Levin's framework, is the distributed representation, encoded in the tissue's bioelectric state, of the organizational configuration the tissue is trying to achieve—the setpoint for anatomical homeostasis toward which cellular behavior is directed (Pezzulo and Levin, 2016; Levin, 2021). It is not a blueprint stored in a nucleus. It is a pattern of membrane potentials maintained across the tissue by the electrical coupling of cells, functioning as a kind of distributed analog memory that encodes the expected organizational state and drives corrective behavior when the current state deviates from it.

This is the informational state in its most concrete biological instantiation. The bioelectric pattern of target morphology is: history-dependent—permanently alterable by physiological experience without any genomic change; distributed—encoded across the entire tissue simultaneously in the pattern of electrical coupling; causally active—governing what individual cells do by constraining which cellular transitions are accessible; and only partially observable—not directly imageable with current clinical technology, though accessible indirectly through impedance imaging. All four properties align exactly with the four properties of the informational state s_t defined in Chapter 9. Target morphology is not an analogy for the informational state. It is one of its concrete biological instantiations.

Cancer as Loss of Bioelectric Coherence

The connection from developmental biology to oncology is direct, and it has been developed most fully in the synthesis between Levin's bioelectric framework and the evolutionary perspective of Davies and Lineweaver (Davies and Lineweaver, 2011; Levin, 2021).

Normal tissue maintains its organizational integrity through bioelectric coherence—the tissue-wide electrical field that coordinates cellular behavior toward collective anatomical goals. Individual cells receive information from this field about where they are in the tissue, what structures surround them, and what behaviors are appropriate to their position within the whole. The bioelectric field is the medium through which the tissue-level organizational state exerts its governance over individual cellular behavior. It is the physical substrate of top-down causation in living tissue.

Cancer, on this view, is fundamentally a disruption of this bioelectric coherence. When the electrical connectivity of cells is corrupted—when the bioelectric field that maintains tissue organization breaks down—cells lose access to the global organizational information that keeps them working toward shared anatomical goals. They revert to more autonomous, more local modes of behavior: proliferating according to their own cellular programs, following gradients that serve individual cellular fitness rather than tissue-level coherence, invading adjacent territories that the organizational field would normally mark as belonging to a different structure.

The disruption is physically measurable. Tumor cells show characteristic depolarization—their resting membrane potential shifts toward zero—and this depolarization disrupts their ability to participate in the tissue-wide bioelectric signaling that maintains organizational coherence (Levin, 2021; Tuszynski et al., 2022). Critically, the depolarization is not merely a consequence of malignant transformation. It is a causal contributor to it.

Artificially depolarizing otherwise normal cells—cells with intact genomes and no oncogenic mutations—can induce metastatic behavior: hyperproliferation, invasion of blood vessels and neural tissue, loss of positional identity (Lobikin et al., 2012). The genetic hardware is normal. The bioelectric organizational state has been corrupted. And the outcome—behavior indistinguishable from malignancy—follows from the state, not from the genome.

Conversely, artificially hyperpolarizing oncogene-bearing cells—restoring their membrane potential toward normal even while the oncogenic mutation remains present and active—can suppress tumor formation. The oncogene is expressed. The oncogenic protein is present. The cell's genomic program for malignant transformation is intact. But the restored bioelectric state overrides it, maintaining the cell within the organizational constraints that define normal tissue behavior (Chernet and Levin, 2014).

These results establish, experimentally and unambiguously, that the organizational state of a tissue—its bioelectric configuration—can override genetic programming in determining biological outcomes. This is top-down causation of the strongest kind operating in real biological tissue. The same conclusion that Chapter 9 established through theoretical argument is here established through experiment.

The Davies-Lineweaver synthesis places this in an evolutionary context. Cancer, they argue, represents a partial reactivation of evolutionarily ancient cellular programs—programs that predate multicellular cooperation, in which cellular fitness and organismal fitness were one and the same

(Davies and Lineweaver, 2011). The bioelectric field that maintains tissue coherence is the mechanism through which multicellular organisms suppress these ancient programs. When that field fails, the ancient programs reassert themselves. The full connection to the atavistic theory and its implications for treatment strategy is developed in Appendix C. What matters here: cancer is not merely a disease of mutant molecules. It is a disease of organizational disruption—instantiated in, and potentially reversible through, the bioelectric state of the tissue.

What the Informational State Is Physically Made Of

The informational state s_t is physically instantiated across multiple organizational layers of the tumor simultaneously. The bioelectric field—the spatial pattern of membrane potentials maintained across the tumor through gap junctional coupling—is one concrete component, encoding the history of prior conditions, the current organizational mode, and the constraints governing which future configurations are accessible. But it is not the only component. The epigenetic landscape encodes another dimension, reflecting the history of prior exposures and constraining which gene expression patterns are currently accessible (Flavahan et al., 2017). The configuration of the gene regulatory network—which feedback loops are active, which bistable switches are in which state—encodes another. The spatial distribution of phenotypic states across the tumor—the clonal architecture shaped by prior selective pressure, the microenvironmental organization produced by vascular and immune history—encodes another still.

The informational state s_t is all of these simultaneously—the full organizational configuration of the tumor across all these layers in their current state as shaped by the entire prior history of the system. Each layer constrains the others. The whole is a coupled, multi-layer organizational configuration that determines what the tumor can become, and it is this whole—not any individual layer—that constitutes the informational state. No single measurement accesses it fully. Each accesses one projection. This is why the Observability Rule is fundamental.

Can the Informational State Be Observed?

Partially, and indirectly—which is a more useful answer than it might initially appear.

No current clinical technology directly images the bioelectric organizational state of a tumor with sufficient spatial resolution to characterize its informational configuration. What can be observed are the consequences of the organizational state on measurable tumor dynamics. This is the principle underlying the TCI framework (Appendix A and B). If the tumor's organizational connectivity is intact—if the informational state is coherent and coupled across the tumor—then the dynamics of different tumor regions will be non-independent. Knowing the state of one region will improve prediction of adjacent regions. TCI quantifies exactly this: the predictive gain from incorporating spatial information into models of tumor dynamics. A high TCI indicates strong organizational coupling consistent with a coherent informational state. A low TCI indicates fragmented dynamics consistent with disrupted organizational coherence.

This is not a direct measurement of the bioelectric state. But it is a principled, falsifiable, quantitative signature of the organizational property that the bioelectric state encodes—visible through the lens of predictive observability, sufficient for principled decision-making under uncertainty as Chapter 13 will show.

Can the Informational State Be Deliberately Manipulated?

The most clinically consequential answer this chapter provides is to this third question, and it is cautiously affirmative.

The planarian experiments establish proof of principle that bioelectric organizational states can be deliberately altered through physiological interventions that do not require changing the genetic sequence. A brief perturbation of gap junctional connectivity permanently rewrites the target morphology. Targeted manipulation of specific ion channels redirects regenerative outcomes. Restoration of normal membrane potential suppresses malignant behavior even in the presence of oncogenic mutations.

These demonstrations are in model organisms, not in clinical tumors undergoing radiotherapy. The gap between proof of principle in planaria and clinical application in human cancer is substantial and should not be minimized. Independent validation at every step is required before any therapeutic claim can be made.

Within the AIG-ART framework developed in Part IV, bioelectric modulation represents an additional dimension of the action space—alongside temporal sequencing, spatial fractionation, and dose magnitude—through which the system's informational state can be perturbed and guided. The machine envisioned in Chapter 16 does not simply deliver radiation in optimized patterns. It acts on the tumor's informational state through every available dimension simultaneously. Bioelectric modulation, as the biology of this chapter establishes, is one such dimension, currently at the proof-of-principle stage but grounded in a biological reality that the framework correctly anticipates.

A conceptual caveat is necessary here. The proposal that an externally applied bioelectric field can selectively modulate tumour coupling while sparing adjacent normal tissue assumes that tumour and normal tissue respond differently to the same applied field. The biological basis for this assumption is the membrane potential differential: depolarized tumour cells and polarized normal cells have measurably different impedance characteristics and gap junctional conductance responses to alternating fields across the frequency spectrum relevant to clinical application. In principle this differential provides a mechanism for tissue selectivity. In practice the quantitative magnitude of the differential, its consistency across tumour types, and its spatial precision at the tumour-normal tissue boundary have not been established experimentally at the tissue level in vivo. The bioelectric field dimension is therefore presented here as a framework-derived prediction—a consequence of the organizational state architecture that is biologically plausible and experimentally testable—rather than as an established therapeutic modality. The experiment required to validate or refute it is specified in Appendix D, prediction T2.4.

The Ghost Has a Body

The ghost in the cancer, introduced in the Preface as something unseen, was given a formal identity in Chapter 9 as the informational state s_t. This chapter has given it a body—a physical instantiation in the tumor's bioelectric organizational field, its epigenetic landscape, its gene regulatory network configuration, and its spatial architecture of phenotypic states.

It is not supernatural. It is not beyond measurement in principle—only beyond current clinical measurement in practice, in the same way that the genome was beyond measurement a century ago, and in the same way that protein structures were beyond resolution before cryo-electron microscopy. It is not static—it evolves continuously under treatment, adapting in ways that reflect both the physics of radiation and the biology of organizational memory and selection. And it is not beyond influence—the experimental record establishes that organizational states can be deliberately altered through physiological means, without editing the genome.

The theoretical framework has its architecture. The biology has its grounding. Three questions have been answered. What remains is to build the machinery through which the informational state—partially observable, causally active, distributed, and evolving—can be tracked, inferred, and used to guide treatment.

That begins with the rules that govern how the state behaves. Chapter 11 develops them.

CHAPTER

11

The Six Rules of Informational-State Radiobiology

A framework without principles, however, is not yet a theory. To generate predictions—to produce expectations that can be tested, compared against observation, and potentially falsified—the informational state framework must be expressed as a set of rules that constrain how the state behaves, how it evolves, and what it implies for response to radiotherapy.

This chapter develops six such rules. Before stating them, one epistemic distinction must be made—because the rules do not all carry the same level of evidential support, and the difference matters for how the framework should be received.

Rules 1 and 2—the State Rule and the History Rule—follow from the observational failures documented in Part I and the identifiability arguments of Chapter 6. Any system producing the pattern of failures across FLASH, SFRT, and SBRT must possess some form of history-dependent internal state. This conclusion rests on mathematical structure rather than on any specific biological model; it would be difficult to avoid without rejecting the observational evidence itself.

Rules 3 through 6—the Constraint Rule, the Interaction Rule, the Nonlinearity Rule, and the Observability Rule—characterise what this framework proposes that state to be: causally active through constraints on component behaviour, spatially and temporally distributed, nonlinear in its dynamics, and only partially observable. These are framework-level claims, supported by the biological evidence of Part II (bioelectric memory in model organisms, associative learning in non-neural systems, phenotypic state transitions without genomic change) and reproduced by the equations of Appendix B under controlled simulation. They are not established in clinical tumours, and Appendix D specifies the experiments that would confirm or revise them.

Both sets of rules are load-bearing for the AIG-ART architecture. But they are not equally established. Rules 1 and 2 describe what must exist for the observational record to make sense. Rules 3 through 6 describe the specific form this book proposes the state takes. Readers who accept Rules 1 and 2 but remain agnostic about 3 through 6 are in a consistent position; they should regard the remainder of this book as a proposal to be tested, not a conclusion to be accepted

Rule 1—The State Rule

> ***"Radiobiological response is governed by the tumor's informational state s_t, not by observable inputs alone."***

This is the foundational rule, the one from which all others flow. It asserts that dose—the variable at the center of conventional radiobiology—is insufficient to determine biological response. What determines response is the combination of the applied input and the organizational state of the system at the time the input is applied.

In formal terms: if R denotes response and D denotes delivered dose, the conventional model assumes $R = f(D)$. The State Rule replaces this with $R = f(D, s_t)$—a function of both dose and state. This is not a minor modification. It changes the nature of the prediction problem from a calculation to an inference. In the conventional model, predicting response requires knowing D. In the state-dependent model, predicting response requires knowing both D and s_t—and since s_t is only partially observable, prediction is inherently probabilistic. The full generalized formulation, in which the classical LQ model is recovered as a special case when s_t is constant and interaction terms vanish, is developed in Appendix A.

The observational grounding is direct across all three anomalies of Part I. FLASH demonstrates that identical total doses produce different responses depending on delivery rate—which, as Chapter 2 established, reveals that the system's state during delivery modulates the effect of each dose increment. SBRT demonstrates that identical doses produce highly variable outcomes across patients whose measured molecular properties are similar—variability that reflects differences in informational state not captured by current measurements. SFRT demonstrates that the same total dose distributed differently in space produces different outcomes—because spatial distribution alters how the state is perturbed and how perturbations propagate through the coupled system.

In each case, dose is held constant while response varies. The State Rule names what accounts for the variation. If response depends on state, then treatment optimization must account for state—which is the inference and control problem that Parts III and IV develop.

Rule 2—The History Rule

> ***"The informational state integrates the tumor's prior exposure. Response depends on the trajectory the system has followed, not only its current position in state space."***

The State Rule establishes that s_t matters. The History Rule specifies how s_t is formed. The organizational state at any time t reflects not only the current condition of the system but the accumulated influence of all prior states—all prior treatments, all prior adaptive responses, all prior transitions. The state is path-dependent. It carries the past forward, encoding it as organizational structure rather than as explicit records.

Formally, this means the state evolves according to a dynamical equation: $s_{t+1} = g(s_t, a_t, \omega_t)$, where a_t is the applied action and ω_t represents stochastic fluctuations. The current state is a function of the previous state and the action taken—meaning the full history of actions shapes the trajectory of states. This equation, and the conditions under which it can be estimated from clinical data, is developed in Appendix A.

The observational grounding is sharpest in the temporal domain. Chapter 2 documented that the order of pulse delivery in FLASH experiments changes outcomes even when total dose and average dose rate are identical—the biological state produced by early pulses is the state within which later pulses act, and this path-dependence is the fingerprint of the History Rule. The M-ROD framework (Appendix A) demonstrates this concretely: time-ordering sensitivity emerges directly from the state evolution equation, not from any separately postulated mechanism.

The History Rule also provides the formal basis for the resistance-as-inference dynamic—now formalised here in the language of the informational state. Each treatment fraction provides information to the tumor system. The state integrates that information—evolving under the selective pressure each fraction applies. After many fractions, the state reflects what the system has learned about the treatment being applied. This is resistance, stated in the language of the History Rule: the state has evolved to a configuration in which the applied treatment produces diminished response, because the system has been guided by the history of prior fractions toward configurations that survive it.

Treatment decisions must therefore account for the full history of prior interventions. A state receptive to a particular action at fraction one may be in an entirely different configuration by fraction ten.

Rule 3—The Constraint Rule

> ***"The informational state governs component-level dynamics by constraining the space of possible transitions. Organizational structure is causally active—top-down causation operates in tumor biology."***

Rules 1 and 2 establish that the state exists and evolves. Rule 3 establishes what the state does—how it exerts its causal influence. The answer, developed theoretically in Chapter 9 and demonstrated biologically in Chapter 10, is through constraints. The informational state does not direct the system's components explicitly. It defines the landscape within which local dynamics unfold—specifying which transitions are accessible and which are not, which configurations are stable and which are unstable, which trajectories the system can follow and which are effectively blocked.

This is top-down causation in the precise sense of Ellis (2012): the higher-level organizational state sets boundary conditions and constraints within which lower-level component behavior operates. The biological grounding for this claim is the experimental record of Chapter 10. Artificially depolarizing genetically normal cells induces malignant behavior. Artificially hyperpolarizing oncogene-bearing cells suppresses malignant behavior despite the continued presence of the oncogenic protein. The organizational state overrides the genetic program—governing what the components do, not by changing the components but by changing the constraints within which they operate.

This is the Constraint Rule demonstrated at its most direct: the same molecular hardware, in different organizational states, produces different biological outcomes. The organizational state is doing causal work that no component-level account can reproduce. For the AIG-ART inference engine, this means maintaining a representation of the state as an organizational entity—a probability distribution over possible organizational configurations—not as a list of molecular parameters.

Rule 4—The Interaction Rule

> ***"The informational state is distributed across the tumor. Its components interact across space and time, so effects are not additive and tumor regions are not independent."***

Rules 1 through 3 establish the existence, history-dependence, and causal power of the state. Rule 4 specifies its spatial and temporal structure. The informational state is not a local property of any individual region. It is a collective property of the tumor system as a whole, maintained through the interactions between its components across space and time.

This means two things with direct clinical consequences. First, the informational state at any location reflects not only local conditions but the state of connected regions and their shared history. A perturbation in one region propagates through the state and alters what is possible elsewhere. Second, the effect of an intervention cannot be predicted by summing its local contributions independently. The system's response to a spatially distributed input is not the sum of its responses to each local component separately. The whole is not the sum of its parts, because the interactions between parts generate properties—and constraints—that the parts do not possess individually.

The observational grounding is SFRT: untreated regions respond to what happens in irradiated regions, in ways that depend on the spatial coupling structure of the system. The proof that conventional scalar metrics are structurally blind to this coupling is established formally in the TCI framework (Appendix A): the mean tumor signal is mathematically invariant under spatial coupling by pairwise symmetry, so two tumors with entirely different coupling structures appear identical in aggregate imaging metrics. The Interaction Rule names why this matters: the coupling is part of the organizational state, and ignoring it means ignoring a causally active dimension of the system.

The bioelectric grounding from Chapter 10 reinforces this directly. Gap junctional connectivity is precisely the mechanism through which organizational information propagates across the tumor as a spatially distributed system. When this connectivity is intact, the tumor behaves as an organized whole. When it is disrupted, regions become more autonomous, more locally driven, and less constrained by the global organizational state. This transition from coupled to fragmented dynamics is what TCI detects—corresponding directly to the biological transition from organized tissue to disorganized malignancy described in Chapter 10. The AIG-ART inference engine must therefore track the state as a spatially distributed object, using voxel-level imaging data interpreted through state-aware models.

Rule 5—The Nonlinearity Rule

> ***"State transitions are nonlinear. The tumor system exhibits thresholds, saturation, and regime transitions that continuous scaling models cannot represent."***

Rule 5 specifies the dynamics of state transitions. The informational state does not change smoothly and proportionally in response to inputs. It changes through nonlinear dynamics that produce qualitatively different behaviors at different scales of perturbation—and this nonlinearity is not a technical complication but a fundamental property of the class of networked biological systems the tumor belongs to.

Below certain thresholds, perturbations produce gradual, roughly proportional responses—the regime in which LQ and related continuous models provide useful approximations. Above those thresholds, perturbations drive the system across bifurcations in state space into qualitatively different configurations. The same input, applied just below and just above a threshold, can produce dramatically different outcomes—not because the biology is different, but because the threshold is a feature of the state space, and crossing it initiates a qualitatively different trajectory.

Three observable signatures follow from the Nonlinearity Rule: threshold behavior—the sharp onset of the FLASH effect above a critical dose rate, the dose-per-fraction threshold beyond which LQ breaks down in SBRT; saturation—the plateauing of the FLASH sparing effect at high dose rates, reflecting the bounded nature of the internal state variable as formalized in M-ROD (Appendix A); and history-dependence of threshold crossing—the same total perturbation crosses different thresholds depending on the state trajectory that preceded it, producing the time-ordering sensitivity documented in Chapter 2.

The bioelectric grounding from Chapter 10 reinforces the Nonlinearity Rule from a different angle. The bistability demonstrated in bioelectric systems—the existence of two stable states corresponding to normal tissue organization and the depolarized malignant configuration—produces precisely the threshold behavior and regime transitions described here. The tumor does not drift gradually from one state to another. It crosses a boundary and lands in a qualitatively different attractor. Resistance, viewed through this lens, is a state transition—crossing a bioelectric bistability threshold into a configuration that is stable against the applied treatment. For AIG-ART, this means more dose is not always better—without state estimation, treatment optimization in a nonlinear state space is navigating blind.

Rule 6—The Observability Rule

> ***"The informational state is only partially observable. Measurements are projections of the state, not the state itself. Inference under uncertainty is therefore***

not a limitation to be overcome but an intrinsic feature of the problem that must be explicitly managed."

Rule 6 completes the logical chain by specifying the epistemic situation of the clinician. The informational state is real, distributed, evolving, and causally active—everything the preceding five rules establish. But it cannot be directly measured. What clinical practice accesses—imaging signals, molecular markers, dose delivery parameters, response assessments—are projections of s_t onto the measurement dimensions that current instruments can reach. These projections carry information about the state, but as the identifiability problem established in Chapter 6, they do not uniquely determine it. Different underlying organizational states can produce identical observable projections. No instrument, however precise, resolves this ambiguity from measurement alone.

This is not a temporary limitation of technology. It is structural—a consequence of the relationship between a high-dimensional organizational state and the low-dimensional observations it produces. What the Observability Rule demands is not better measurement—though better measurement helps—but a different approach to prediction. Instead of attempting to determine the state exactly, which is impossible, the clinician must maintain and update a probability distribution over possible states: the belief state $b_t(s) = p(s_t = s \mid o_1{:}t, a_1{:}t_{-1})$. This belief is not a confession of ignorance. It is the optimal representation of what is known about the state given all available observations and the constraints imposed by the preceding five rules. The full framework for computing and updating this belief is developed in Appendix A and implemented in the AIG-ART architecture of Chapter 16.

The Observability Rule also provides the formal grounding for the most important game-theoretic insight of the book. The tumor is performing its own form of inference—its evolutionary dynamics extracting information from treatment and updating the state toward configurations that survive it. The clinician is performing inference about the tumor—observations updating the belief state and informing the next treatment decision. These two inference processes run in parallel. The outcome of treatment depends on which runs faster and more accurately. This is the strategic logic of AIG-ART: not to deliver the optimal fixed plan, but to play an inference game against an adaptive opponent and win by updating faster.

The Rules as an Integrated System

The six rules form a single logical chain in which each rule follows from the previous and requires what follows: Rule 1 says response depends on state. Rule 2 says state depends on history. Rule 3 says state governs components through constraints. Rule 4 says state is distributed and effects are non-additive. Rule 5 says state transitions are nonlinear. Rule 6 says state is only partially observable.

Remove any link and the chain breaks—without Rule 1 there is no state to reason about; without Rule 6 the inference problem and with it AIG-ART become unnecessary. Together, the six rules define the minimal theoretical structure from which the three anomalies of Part I follow as expected rather than puzzling, from which the biological evidence of Part II is explanatory rather than merely descriptive, and from which the inference and control framework of Part IV is the clinically necessary response.

The framework has its rules. What it needs now is its first measurement instrument—a tool that makes at least one dimension of the hidden state partially visible, that can be computed from data already accessible in clinical MR-guided radiotherapy, and that provides the initial foothold for state-aware treatment decisions.

That instrument is the Tumor Coupling Index. Chapter 12 introduces it.

PART III

Reconstructing the Hidden State of the Tumour

Part II built the framework. It established what the informational state is, why it must exist, what it is physically made of, and what rules govern its behavior. That work was necessarily abstract—you cannot formalize something you haven't first understood.

Part III asks a different question: how do we begin to see it?

Two chapters and one conceptual bridge. The Tumor Coupling Index makes one dimension of the hidden state partially visible from data already being collected in MR-guided radiotherapy. The belief state and free energy framework provide the principled machinery for reasoning under the uncertainty that partial visibility creates. Chapter 14 then closes the loop—returning to the three anomalies of Part I and showing that they are no longer anomalies when read through the framework.

The mathematics in these chapters is real but the book carries the reader through it. What matters most is the conceptual move: from hidden to partially visible, from unknown to probabilistically estimated, from anomaly to expected signature. That move is what makes Part IV possible.

CHAPTER

12

Detecting Structure: The Tumor Coupling Index

The six rules of Chapter 11 define the informational state framework with theoretical precision. But a framework that cannot make contact with measurement—that remains entirely in the space of organizational abstractions—is not yet useful clinically. At some point, the hidden must become partially visible. The organizational state that governs tumor behavior must leave traces in data that clinicians can actually collect. And those traces must be detectable by methods that do not require perfect knowledge of the underlying state—that work, as clinical tools must, from incomplete and noisy observations.

This chapter introduces the first such tool.

It addresses a specific problem that emerges directly from the Interaction Rule: the tumor's spatial coupling—the degree to which different regions interact and influence each other's dynamics—is a real and causally relevant feature of the informational state, but it is invisible to the scalar imaging metrics that dominate current clinical practice. Two tumors with entirely different internal coupling structures can produce identical mean ADC trajectories, identical volumetric responses, identical aggregate imaging signatures. The coupling is there. The conventional measurement cannot see it.

The question is whether a different kind of measurement can.

The Blind Spot in Current Imaging

The argument that conventional metrics are blind to spatial coupling is not intuitive, but it is mathematically precise and worth stating clearly.

Consider a tumor modeled as a collection of voxels, each characterized by an imaging-derived signal—the apparent diffusion coefficient from diffusion-weighted MRI, for example. In a spatially independent tumor, each voxel evolves according to its own local dynamics, without influence from its neighbors. In a coupled tumor, each voxel's evolution depends partly on the states of adjacent voxels—information propagates across the tumor, and regions influence each other.

Now ask: what does the mean ADC signal across all voxels do in each case? The coupling term in any physically reasonable spatial model takes the form of a discrete Laplacian—each voxel is pushed toward the average of its neighbors, redistributing values across the tumor without changing their sum. When you take the mean across all voxels, this redistribution term cancels by pairwise symmetry: every transfer from voxel i to voxel j is exactly offset by the corresponding term from j to i. The mean evolves according to local dynamics only—exactly as it would if the coupling were absent (Appendix A and B).

The mathematical consequence is stark: the mean ADC trajectory is independent of the coupling strength. A tumor in which every region influences every neighbor produces identical mean ADC curves to one in which every region evolves in complete isolation. Volumetric measures, aggregate response metrics, any summary statistic that averages across the tumor—all are structurally blind to spatial coupling, not as a matter of measurement precision but as a matter of mathematical necessity.

To detect coupling, a completely different analytical strategy is required—not a new imaging acquisition, but a new question asked of the same data.

Structure Reveals Itself Through Prediction

The key insight that makes the Tumor Coupling Index possible is this: while coupling is invisible to conventional metrics, it has a specific and detectable consequence for the system's predictive structure. If tumor regions are coupled—if the state of one region genuinely influences the future state of its neighbors—then knowing the current state of neighboring regions should improve prediction of any given region's future state. If regions are independent, knowing the neighbors adds nothing to prediction beyond what the region's own current state provides.

This shifts the detection problem from a question about parameters to a question about prediction. Instead of asking "what is the coupling parameter?"—which requires solving an inverse problem that is both ill-posed and assumption-laden—we ask "does including spatial information improve prediction?" The answer is measurable directly from data, without specifying any particular model of the coupling mechanism, without estimating any unobservable parameters, and without making strong assumptions about the biological processes that generate the coupling.

This approach connects to a tradition in statistics and information theory where causal structure is inferred through improvements in prediction. Granger causality—the principle that X causes Y if knowing X's history improves prediction of Y's future beyond what Y's own history provides—is the canonical example (Granger, 1969). Transfer entropy extends this to nonlinear systems (Schreiber, 2000). The TCI framework applies a structurally similar principle to the spatial domain of tumor imaging: spatial coupling is inferred from the spatial predictive advantage, not from explicit parameter estimation.

Defining the Tumor Coupling Index

The formal definition follows from this predictive principle (Appendix A).

Two predictive models are constructed from the same longitudinal ADC data that scalar metrics fail to exploit—the voxel-level apparent diffusion coefficient time series acquired at each treatment fraction through serial diffusion-weighted

MRI. The first—the independent model—predicts the future ADC of each voxel using only that voxel's own current and recent history. The second—the spatial model—predicts the future ADC of each voxel using both its own history and the current ADC values of its spatial neighbors. Both models are fit to the observed data. Both are evaluated on their prediction error.

The Tumor Coupling Index is defined as the normalized reduction in prediction error achieved by the spatial model relative to the independent model:

$$\mathrm{TCI} = \frac{E_{\mathrm{ind}} - E_{\mathrm{spatial}}}{E_{\mathrm{ind}}}$$

where E_ind is the mean squared prediction error of the independent model and E_spatial is the mean squared prediction error of the spatial model. The normalization ensures TCI is dimensionless and interpretable across different tumors and imaging protocols.

The interpretation is direct. When TCI ≈ 0, the spatial model provides no predictive advantage over the independent model—the tumor's regions evolve without meaningful influence from their neighbors, consistent with organizational fragmentation and low coupling. When TCI > 0, the spatial model predicts better—knowing the ADC state of neighboring regions genuinely improves prediction of future states, which is only possible if those regions are informationally connected, if the organizational state is propagating across the tumor in a way that creates predictive structure.

TCI does not identify the biological mechanism of coupling. It does not estimate a coupling parameter. It detects the observable consequence of coupling—the predictive advantage conferred by spatial ADC information—and quantifies it as a single, interpretable number.

What the Simulations Show

The behavior of TCI under controlled conditions was established through simulation studies in which the presence and strength of spatial coupling could be specified exactly, allowing the metric's sensitivity and specificity to be assessed against a known ground truth (Appendix A and B).

Under independent dynamics—no spatial coupling—TCI remains near zero across multiple independent simulations. The spatial model provides no consistent predictive advantage when none exists. This is the null behavior that any valid detection metric must satisfy: it should not produce false positives, should not detect structure in independent systems, should not create the appearance of coupling from noise alone.

When spatial coupling is introduced at any nonzero strength, TCI rises substantially and clearly separates from the null distribution. The separation spans multiple orders of magnitude in the simulated systems, with no overlap between the distributions of TCI under independence and under coupling. The metric detects real structure reliably.

When the temporal or spatial structure of the data is destroyed—by randomly permuting the ADC time series of each voxel, or by randomly shuffling voxel locations at each time point—TCI collapses back to near-zero values. This falsifiability check is critical: it confirms that TCI is responding to genuine spatiotemporal structure in the ADC data, not to statistical artifacts or incidental correlations that would survive randomization.

As coupling strength increases from weak to strong, TCI increases monotonically—providing a continuous, quantitative measure of how strongly the tumor's regions interact, rather than a binary classification of coupled versus uncoupled. This graded response means TCI carries information not just about whether coupling exists but about how strong it is, which is essential for its role as a structural prior in the state estimation framework.

What TCI Is Measuring—and What It Is Not

TCI measures the observable consequence of spatial interaction—the predictive advantage conferred by incorporating spatial ADC information into models of tumor dynamics. It does not measure a specific biological parameter. It does not identify which mechanism is generating the coupling—whether bystander effects, bioelectric field propagation, immune signaling, or vascular microenvironmental gradients. Any mechanism that causes the future ADC of a voxel to depend on the current ADC of its neighbors will produce a positive TCI. The metric is mechanism-agnostic by design—a strength in the clinical context where biological mechanisms are numerous, entangled, and in many cases unresolvable from imaging data alone.

What TCI is not: it is not a measure of tumor malignancy, prognosis, or treatment response in the conventional sense. It is a measure of organizational structure—specifically, the degree to which the tumor's different regions are informationally connected, the degree to which the informational state is distributed and coherent across the tumor rather than fragmented into independent regional dynamics. Whether high TCI is good or bad in any particular clinical context depends on how that organizational structure interacts with the specific treatment being applied—a question the AIG-ART framework addresses in Part IV.

TCI Within the Informational State Framework

Within the six rules of Chapter 11, TCI occupies a specific and important position. It is a partial observable of the Interaction Rule—providing a quantitative signature of the distributional and coupling properties of the informational state that Rule 4 establishes as causally relevant.

Rule 4 asserts that the state is distributed and that effects are not additive because regions interact. TCI measures how strongly this interaction manifests in observable ADC dynamics. A high TCI is evidence that Rule 4 is operating with significant force—that the tumor's organizational state is actively coupling its regions, propagating perturbations across space, and producing collective dynamics that cannot be predicted from independent regional ADC models. A low TCI suggests that regions are behaving more autonomously, consistent with reduced organizational coherence and a more fragmented informational state.

Within the AIG-ART inference architecture, TCI functions as a structural prior that constrains the belief state $b_t(s)$. The organizational coupling that TCI detects eliminates certain organizational configurations from the belief distribution—configurations in which regions evolve independently are inconsistent with a high TCI, and vice versa. This constraint narrows the range of possible states consistent with observations, improving the precision of state estimation and the reliability of subsequent treatment decisions. The formal integration of TCI into the belief state update is developed in Appendix A. Chapter 14 develops how TCI guides the selection of probing modality—which delivery structure will generate the most informative response given the current coupling estimate.

A Clinical Window Into Organizational State

The introduction of TCI marks a transition in the book's argument. Through Chapters 6 to 11, the informational state was developed theoretically and grounded biologically, but it remained inaccessible to measurement. TCI changes this, partially. Two tumors that appear identical in conventional imaging—identical mean ADC, identical volume, identical response rate—may have very different TCI values, reflecting very different degrees of organizational coupling. Those differences are not noise. They are signal—signal about the organizational state that will determine how the tumor responds to spatially structured interventions, how it propagates perturbations, and how its evolutionary dynamics will unfold under treatment pressure.

The clinical context for TCI is MR-guided radiotherapy, where serial diffusion-weighted imaging is acquired at every treatment fraction as a matter of routine. This longitudinal, voxel-level ADC data stream is precisely what TCI requires—and it is the same data that, when collapsed into mean trajectories, is mathematically blind to the coupling that TCI detects. The mean ADC fails as a coupling metric not because it lacks data but because averaging destroys the spatial predictive structure that coupling creates. TCI recovers that structure by asking not what the average ADC does, but whether knowing one voxel's ADC improves prediction of its neighbours'. A different analysis of the same acquisition, producing a categorically different kind of information.

TCI is a measurement instrument, not the framework itself. Its failure would indicate that serial ADC dynamics lack sufficient sensitivity or specificity to detect spatial organisational coupling at clinically relevant resolutions—a measurement limitation, not a theoretical one. The informational state is established independently through the biological evidence of Chapters 8 and 10 and the mathematical necessity argued in Chapter 6. Other instruments—EIT, photoacoustic oxygen dynamics, direct bioelectric imaging—access different projections of the same underlying state. TCI failure would mean we need a better window. It would not mean there is nothing to see.

From Detection to Inference

TCI provides one observable dimension of the informational state. Treatment response itself—how the tumor responds to each fraction, whether it matches prediction or surprises—is informative about the state. The evolution of TCI over successive fractions is informative in its own right: a TCI that rises during treatment suggests growing organizational coherence, a fingerprint of a system learning its treatment rather than merely responding to it; one that falls suggests progressive organizational disruption consistent with effective state perturbation. Each observation constrains the belief distribution over possible states and leads to better-informed subsequent decisions.

Before the inference and control framework can be built, one more conceptual piece must be established: the formal relationship between hidden state, partial observability, uncertainty, and the principled framework for reasoning under that uncertainty.

That is the subject of Chapter 13.

CHAPTER

13

From Hidden State to Uncertainty and Free Energy

Knowing that the state exists, knowing that it governs behavior, knowing that it can be partially detected—none of this tells us how to form beliefs about the state from incomplete observations, how to update those beliefs as new data arrives, or how to choose actions that account for what we do not know. That framework is what this chapter builds.

It is the conceptual engine of the book. Everything in Part IV—the AIG-ART architecture, the probing strategy, the game-theoretic treatment policy—runs on it.

The Nature of the Problem

Begin with the clinical situation as it actually is, stripped of the comfortable fictions that conventional planning imports.

A patient arrives for their fifth fraction of radiotherapy. You have imaging from four prior fractions—ADC dynamics, TCI trajectory, treatment responses. You have the treatment history: what was delivered, when, at what dose rate, in what spatial pattern. What you do not have—what you cannot have, for reasons established across Chapters 6, 9, and 12—is knowledge of the tumor's informational state. The imaging gives you projections. The TCI gives you one organizational property. But the state itself—the full organizational configuration of the tumor, the bioelectric field pattern, the epigenetic landscape, the clonal architecture, the configuration of regulatory networks—is not accessible to direct measurement. Multiple different underlying states are consistent with everything you can observe.

In this situation, the clinician faces a choice. One option is to pretend the uncertainty does not exist—to treat the observed variables as though they fully determined the state, to plan the next fraction as though the system were fully known. This is what conventional radiotherapy does, and it is why the outcomes documented in Part I are so resistant to explanation: the plan is optimized for a system that is assumed to be known, when the system is in fact only partially observable. The other option is to acknowledge the uncertainty explicitly, represent it formally, and make it the basis for principled decision-making. This is what the framework developed in this chapter does.

Belief Over State

If the informational state s_t cannot be directly known, the appropriate representation of what is known about it is not a single estimate but a probability distribution—a spread of plausible states, each associated with a degree of credibility given everything that has been observed and done.

This distribution is called the belief state:

$b_t(s) = p(s_t = s \mid o_1{:}t, a_1{:}t_{-1})$

Read in plain language: the belief at time t is the probability that the system is in organizational configuration s, given all observations o_1 through o_t and all actions a_1 through a_{t-1} taken up to the current moment. It is the clinician's best current assessment of where in state space the tumor is—not a point estimate, but a full distribution over possibilities.

This is not a statistical technicality. It is the correct representation of the clinician's epistemic situation. Every piece of information—each imaging acquisition, each observed treatment response, each TCI measurement—shifts this distribution, sharpening it around states consistent with the observation and diminishing the credibility of states inconsistent with it. The belief state is a living summary of everything known about the tumor's organizational configuration, updated continuously as new data arrives.

TCI enters here as a structural constraint on the belief state. A measured TCI value—say, a moderately high value suggesting significant spatial coupling—eliminates from the belief distribution all organizational configurations in which tumor regions behave independently. It does not uniquely determine the state. But it narrows the range of plausible states substantially, making some configurations much more credible and others effectively ruled out. The formal mechanism by which TCI constrains the belief state is developed in Appendix A.

Uncertainty Is Not the Enemy

There is a tendency in clinical medicine to treat uncertainty as a failure—as something to be eliminated by more measurement, better imaging, or deeper molecular profiling. The framework developed here takes a different position. Uncertainty, in a partially observable system, is not a failure. It is information about the limits of what can be known. And managed correctly—represented explicitly, updated principally, incorporated into decision-making—it is more useful than a false certainty that ignores the limits of observation.

The belief state is the mechanism through which uncertainty is managed rather than suppressed. It tells the clinician not only what the most likely state is, but how confident that estimate is—how broad or narrow the distribution is, how much different plausible states would diverge in their response to the proposed next action. A narrow belief distribution means relatively confident state estimation—different plausible states will respond similarly to the same action. A broad belief distribution means high uncertainty—different plausible states could respond very differently, and the choice of action matters more.

This distinction drives one of the most important insights of the framework: in high-uncertainty situations, the optimal action may not be the one that maximizes expected tumor control under the current belief. It may be the one that most effectively reduces uncertainty—that perturbs the system in a way that generates an informative response, sharpening the belief distribution and enabling better decisions in subsequent fractions. Treatment and measurement are not separate activities. They are coupled, and the coupling must be made explicit in the decision framework.

The Free Energy Principle

At this point a deeper question arises. The belief state provides the representation. But what governs the process of belief updating and action selection? What is the principled framework that connects observations to belief updates, and belief states to treatment decisions?

The answer that this book adopts—and that connects the radiotherapy problem to a much broader framework in theoretical neuroscience and statistical physics—is the Free Energy Principle (Friston et al., 2017).

The Free Energy Principle proposes that self-organizing biological systems behave in ways that minimize a quantity called variational free energy—a measure of the discrepancy between the system's internal model of the world and the observations it receives. Minimizing free energy is equivalent, in the limit of a perfect model, to Bayesian belief updating: the system updates its internal representation to bring it into alignment with observations, reducing surprise.

What makes the FEP more than just a restatement of Bayesian inference is its extension to action. Under the FEP, systems do not only update their internal models to reduce free energy—they also act on their environment to bring observations into alignment with predictions, further reducing free energy. This is active inference: perception and action are coupled aspects of a single process of free energy minimization, not separate systems operating in sequence.

For the AIG-ART framework, the FEP provides three things. First, a principled account of how the belief state should be updated—through variational Bayesian inference that minimizes the discrepancy between predicted and observed states. Second, a principled account of how actions should be selected—by minimizing expected free energy over the distribution of possible future states, balancing the reduction of uncertainty (epistemic value) against the achievement of desired outcomes (extrinsic value). Third, a natural account of clinical conservatism—the complexity cost term in the free energy decomposition penalizes actions that deviate substantially from prior expectations, providing an automatic brake against aggressive interventions under high uncertainty. The full mathematical derivation of variational free energy and its decomposition into these three components is given in Appendix A.

Free Energy Minimization and Resistance

Here the framework delivers its deepest insight—the one that connects the physics of inference to the biology of treatment failure.

The tumor is also a system. And like any biological system that persists and adapts, it behaves in ways consistent with the Free Energy Principle. Under treatment, the tumor experiences massive surprise—radiation produces conditions radically inconsistent with the organizational states the tumor has been maintaining. The tumor's evolutionary and adaptive dynamics respond in exactly the way the FEP predicts: they update the internal configuration—the informational state—to bring it into better alignment with the treatment environment, and they act on the microenvironment to make that environment less threatening.

Resistance is free energy minimization. It is the tumor's organizational dynamics reducing their own surprise—updating the state toward configurations that are no longer shocked by the applied treatment, and acting on the microenvironment through secreted signals, vascular remodeling, and immune evasion to bring the treatment's effects into alignment with what the current state can tolerate.

This formulation is not a metaphor. It is a mathematical claim: the tumor's adaptive dynamics under selective pressure are formally equivalent to an inference process, updating a distribution over viable configurations in response to treatment-as-evidence, converging on states that minimize the free energy generated by the applied intervention (Friston et al., 2017; Harper, 2009).

The clinical implication is now stated with maximum precision. A fixed treatment policy—the same dose, the same fractionation, the same delivery structure, repeated identically—is a stationary source of surprise. The tumor's adaptive inference will find it, learn its structure, and evolve toward configurations that are no longer surprised by it. This is resistance as completed inference. The solution is not to apply more of the same policy with greater intensity—that merely accelerates the inference, giving the tumor more evidence under greater selective pressure. The solution is to make the treatment policy non-stationary—to change it faster than the tumor's adaptive dynamics can converge. This is the game-theoretic logic of AIG-ART: not to find the optimal fixed strategy, but to play an adaptive game in which the clinician's policy evolves faster than the tumor's state can converge on a resistant configuration.

The clinician minimizes free energy about the tumor's state—updating the belief state with each new observation, reducing uncertainty about where in state space the tumor currently is. The tumor minimizes free energy about the treatment—updating its organizational state to reduce the surprise generated by each fraction. Both are inference processes. The one that updates faster wins.

The POMDP: Formalizing the Problem

The problem now has a formal name in the literature of decision theory and artificial intelligence: a Partially Observable Markov Decision Process, or POMDP (Kaelbling et al., 1998).

A POMDP describes exactly the situation we face. There is a system with a hidden state that evolves over time according to dynamics influenced by the actions taken. Observations are generated by the state but do not uniquely determine it. The decision-maker maintains a belief over possible states, updated by Bayesian inference as observations arrive. Actions are selected to maximize expected outcomes over the distribution of possible states—accounting for both the therapeutic effect and the informational value of different actions.

In the radiotherapy POMDP, the hidden state is the tumor's informational state s_t. The observations are imaging data, TCI values, and treatment responses. The actions are the treatment decisions—dose magnitude, delivery rate, spatial fractionation pattern, temporal sequencing, particle type. The dynamics are the state evolution equation of Rule 2. The belief state is $b_t(s)$. The objective is to select a sequence of actions that guides the tumor's state toward desired configurations—tumor control, reduced resistance—while managing the uncertainty about which state the tumor is currently in.

The solution to a POMDP is a policy—a mapping from belief states to actions—not a fixed plan. The policy specifies what to do given the current belief, whatever that belief turns out to be. It is adaptive by construction: as the belief state changes in response to new observations, the recommended action changes with it. This is what makes AIG-ART fundamentally different from conventional adaptive radiotherapy, which adapts to geometric changes in tumor anatomy but does not adapt to inferred changes in the tumor's organizational state. The POMDP policy adapts to the state—as estimated, under uncertainty, from all available evidence.

The POMDP specifies a hidden state space over which the clinician maintains a belief, an action space of treatment decisions, a transition model describing how the state evolves under each action, an observation model connecting the hidden state to what the sensing architecture can measure, a reward function encoding the clinical objectives, and a discount factor balancing immediate and future therapeutic goals. Together these six components define the inference and control problem that AIG-ART solves at every treatment fraction.

A related framework—the predictive digital twin approach of Hormuth et al. (2023)—applies Bayesian state estimation to tumour response modelling in high-grade glioma, optimising radiotherapy under uncertainty from serial MRI. That work operates at the level of tumour cell density within a known mechanistic model; the POMDP formulation here operates at the level of the organisational state s_t, which is not directly accessible to any measurement and is not captured by any cell-density model. The distinction is not technical but conceptual: the informational state is not a better-measured version of a known quantity. It is a different kind of object entirely.

Actions as Experiments

One consequence of the POMDP formulation deserves particular emphasis because it changes how each treatment fraction should be understood.

In a fully observed system—one where the state is known—actions are purely interventions. You know the state, you know what action will produce the desired state transition, you apply it. There is no information to be gained from the action, because you already know everything relevant.

In a partially observed system—one where the state is uncertain—actions are simultaneously interventions and experiments. Each action perturbs the system and generates a response. That response is an observation that updates the belief state—and different actions generate different responses, with different informational content about the hidden state.

Some actions may be highly therapeutic but informationally uninformative—producing large expected tumor control regardless of which state the tumor is in, and therefore telling the clinician little about which state it actually occupies. Other actions may be moderately therapeutic but highly informative—producing responses that differ substantially depending on which state the tumor is in, and therefore allowing the clinician to sharpen their belief substantially from the observed response.

The optimal action balances these two considerations. This is the exploitation-exploration tradeoff in the language of reinforcement learning—and in the language of AIG-ART, it is the principle that treatment and measurement are inseparable. Every fraction is both a therapeutic intervention and a probe. The design of the fraction—the choice of dose rate, spatial pattern, fractionation structure, particle type—determines not only what the fraction does to the tumor but what information about the tumor's state it generates.

This is why the three modalities examined in Part I—FLASH, SFRT, SBRT—appear again in Part IV not as separate clinical techniques but as probes of specific dimensions of the hidden state. FLASH probes the temporal sensitivity of the state—the oxygen-memory component formalized in M-ROD. SFRT probes the spatial coupling structure—the organizational connectivity that TCI detects. SBRT probes the nonlinear regime boundaries—the thresholds and bifurcations of the state space that the Nonlinearity Rule describes. Each modality generates a specific kind of information about the state. AIG-ART selects among them—and combines them—based on which will most efficiently reduce uncertainty about the current state while advancing toward the desired therapeutic outcome.

The Expected Free Energy Decomposition

The formal criterion for action selection under the FEP is the minimization of expected free energy G(a)—the free energy expected to arise if action a is taken, averaged over the current belief distribution. This decomposes into three components (Friston et al., 2017; Appendix A):

The first component is extrinsic value—the expected degree to which the action achieves desired outcomes, specifically tumor control and normal tissue sparing. This is the therapeutic objective: drive the tumor toward states associated with good clinical outcomes.

The second component is epistemic value—the expected reduction in uncertainty about the state that the action will generate. Actions that probe the system informationally—that generate responses differentially informative about the state—score highly on this component. This is the informational objective: reduce uncertainty about the state to enable better future decisions.

The third component is complexity cost—the penalty for actions that deviate substantially from prior expectations, providing automatic conservatism under high uncertainty. When the belief distribution is broad—when many different states are plausible—the complexity cost penalizes aggressive actions that would be catastrophic if the tumor is in one plausible state even if optimal in another. This is clinical caution, engineered directly into the decision criterion rather than imposed as an external constraint.

The balance between these three components changes dynamically as the belief state evolves—early in treatment, epistemic value dominates and the policy favors informative probing; as the belief sharpens, extrinsic value takes over and the policy transitions toward aggressive exploitation of the now-better-estimated state. Not a fixed protocol. A dynamic policy that evolves with the belief.

What This Chapter Has Built

Four things that Part IV will use directly: the belief state $b_t(s)$ as the correct representation of the clinician's knowledge; the Free Energy Principle as the normative framework governing both the clinician's inference and the tumor's adaptation—unifying the therapeutic and resistance problems within a single mathematical structure; the POMDP as the formal problem class; and the expected free energy decomposition as the criterion for action selection. With this foundation, Part IV can be built.

The ghost can now be tracked. The question is how to use that tracking to guide the system toward where we want it to go.

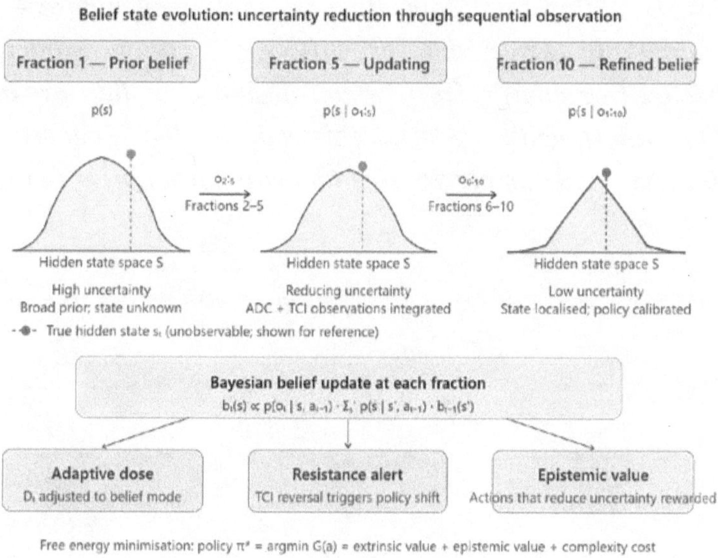

Figure 13.1. *Belief state evolution through sequential observation during a course of radiotherapy. At fraction 1, the belief state $b_t(s)$ is broad—the clinician has limited information about the tumour's hidden organizational state and the prior distribution spans a wide region of state space. As observations accumulate across fractions—ADC dynamics, TCI trajectory, EIT coherence, PET SUV—the Bayesian update equation narrows the belief distribution around the true hidden state (shown in red for reference; unobservable in clinical practice). By fraction 10, the belief state is sharply peaked, enabling a calibrated adaptive policy. Three clinical consequences follow from a refined belief state: dose magnitude can be adjusted to the estimated state, a TCI reversal triggers a resistance interception response, and actions with high epistemic value—those that discriminate*

between closely competing state hypotheses—are preferentially selected. The AIG-ART policy minimises expected free energy G(a), which decomposes into extrinsic value (therapeutic goal), epistemic value (uncertainty reduction), and complexity cost (deviation from prior policy).

CHAPTER

14

Reinterpreting the Anomalies: From Observation to Mechanism

Now it is time to close the loop.

This chapter returns to the three anomalies and reinterprets them—not as mysterious exceptions requiring separate biological explanations, but as expected signatures of a nonlinear, partially observable, history-dependent dynamical system being probed along its three fundamental axes. Each anomaly, viewed through the informational state framework, becomes intelligible. And each, viewed through the AIG-ART lens introduced in Chapter 13, becomes not a problem to be managed but a tool to be used.

The Interpretive Shift

The conventional response to each anomaly has followed a recognisable pattern: identify a plausible mechanism—oxygen depletion for FLASH, bystander signalling for SFRT, vascular damage for SBRT—study it, partially validate it, find it insufficient, propose another. The debate continues. Prediction remains elusive.

This pattern is not accidental. It is the expected outcome of applying a mechanistic, bottom-up explanatory strategy to phenomena that arise from organizational, top-down causation. The mechanisms proposed for each anomaly are real—oxygen depletion does contribute to FLASH, bystander effects do contribute to SFRT, vascular damage does contribute to SBRT. But they are components of the system's response, not its cause.

This is not a claim that mechanistic research is unnecessary—it is a claim about the relationship between levels of description. Mechanistic models specify what the components do: how oxygen is depleted by a radiation pulse, how bystander signals propagate between cells, how vascular architecture responds to high-dose injury.

The informational state specifies the organisational context within which those mechanisms operate: which threshold the system is currently near, how strongly regions are coupled, what trajectory a perturbation will initiate.

Neither level is sufficient without the other. Mechanistic models without an organisational context cannot predict when oxygen depletion will produce dramatic normal tissue sparing and when it will not.

An organisational state without mechanistic grounding has no account of what is physically happening at the cellular level. The generalized radiobiological model, developed in the later sections of this chapter, is the formal expression of this coexistence. The mechanisms are the engine. The informational state is the terrain.

FLASH as Temporal State Probing

FLASH radiotherapy delivers radiation at dose rates exceeding forty Gray per second—orders of magnitude above conventional clinical practice. The biological consequence, documented across multiple tissues and species, is a dramatic reduction in normal tissue toxicity while tumor control is preserved (Favaudon et al., 2014; Vozenin et al., 2019). The delivery time for a therapeutic dose collapses from minutes to milliseconds. And as Chapter 2 documented, the biological response depends not only on the total dose and average dose rate, but on the fine temporal structure of delivery—pulse spacing, duty cycle, irradiation sequence.

In the conventional framework, these temporal dependencies are anomalous. Radiosensitivity should depend on dose and oxygen, not on the microsecond-level pattern of pulse delivery.

In the informational state framework, they are expected. The temporal structure of delivery determines how the internal state variable evolves during irradiation. The state does not respond instantaneously to radiation—it evolves through the dynamics formalized in M-ROD (Appendix A): activation driven by dose rate through a cooperative, threshold-dependent function, reinforced by positive feedback within the state, decaying between pulses at a characteristic timescale, bounded by the finite capacity of the biological system. The radiosensitivity that any given pulse encounters is the radiosensitivity produced by the state that prior pulses have established.

This is why pulse spacing matters. Closely spaced pulses allow the state to accumulate—each pulse building on the activated state left by the previous one, producing higher cumulative activation and therefore greater normal tissue protection. Widely spaced pulses allow the state to decay between pulses—each pulse encounters a less activated state, cumulative protection is reduced, and the FLASH effect diminishes. The same total dose and average dose rate, different temporal structure, different state trajectory, different biological outcome. The History Rule at work in the most direct possible way. Notably, the quantitative consistency analysis in the following section independently supports this picture, lending further credibility to the informational state framework.

The threshold behavior—the sharp onset of FLASH effect above a critical dose rate—reflects the nonlinearity of the state activation function. Below the threshold, the cooperative activation term is insufficient to drive significant state activation. Above it, the system crosses a bifurcation in state space and the activation dynamics take over, driving rapid protection. The Nonlinearity Rule made visible.

The saturation of the FLASH effect at very high dose rates reflects the bounded nature of the state variable—M cannot exceed one, regardless of how high the dose rate goes. The biological system has finite protective capacity. The Constraint Rule and the State Rule together, making a prediction that the M-ROD framework confirms.

And the time-ordering sensitivity—the fact that high-dose-rate pulses delivered first produce different outcomes from the same pulses delivered last—is the purest expression of the History Rule. Path-dependence. The state that the first set of pulses creates is the state in which the second set operates. Change the order, change the state trajectory, change the biological outcome.

The physical substrate that implements these dynamics is the subject of the timescale synthesis in Chapter 15 and the formal model specification in Appendix A; here what matters is that the state exists, evolves, and carries memory—and that these three properties alone are sufficient to reinterpret FLASH's behaviour through the six rules.

FLASH is not a chemical anomaly or a special case. It is a temporal probe of the informational state—a way of driving the state along a specific temporal trajectory and observing what that trajectory produces in terms of differential tissue response. In the AIG-ART framework, FLASH becomes a controlled temporal intervention: a tool for driving the tumor's informational state through a specific temporal trajectory while simultaneously generating observations—the differential response between tumor and normal tissue—that update the belief state and inform subsequent treatment decisions.

A Quantitative Consistency Check for FLASH

The reinterpretation of FLASH above is qualitative—it explains how the anomalies fit into the informational-state framework rather than demonstrating that the framework's quantitative predictions bear scrutiny. One such check is worth performing here, because it is where the framework's ambitions most directly meet the numbers.

The check concerns the fast layer of s_t, formalised as M(t) in the M-ROD model, and asks whether the decay timescale τ_M = 1/γ required by the FLASH phenomenology is consistent with any known biological substrate that could plausibly realise it.

Deriving the required timescale from FLASH phenomenology.

M-ROD's most discriminating prediction, registered as T2.1 in Appendix D, is that FLASH outcomes depend on pulse spacing at fixed total dose and average dose rate—a dependence no memoryless model can produce. For this prediction to be realisable, τ_M must satisfy a specific condition. If τ_M is much shorter than the inter-pulse interval, M decays completely between pulses and each pulse starts from baseline; pulse spacing becomes irrelevant. If τ_M is much longer than the total delivery time, M integrates across all pulses regardless of spacing; again, pulse spacing becomes irrelevant. Pulse-spacing sensitivity exists only when τ_M is comparable to the inter-pulse interval itself.

Modern FLASH accelerators deliver pulses of microsecond to millisecond duration, with inter-pulse intervals ranging from ~2 ms to ~500 ms depending on modality and pulse structure. Numerical simulation of the M-ROD dynamics across this range (reported in Appendix B, with parameters matched to the M-ROD preprint) shows pulse-spacing sensitivity peaking at τ_M ≈ 80 ms and remaining substantial across τ_M ≈ 10 –

200 ms. Below 5 ms, sensitivity falls because M cannot accumulate across pulses. Above 1 s, it falls because M approaches saturation regardless of spacing.

The framework therefore predicts:

$$\tau\_M \approx 10 - 100 \text{ ms}$$

This prediction is independent of the Hill function parameters that set the dose-rate threshold (K, n), and independent of the activation rate α_M. It comes specifically from the requirement that pulse-spacing sensitivity be observable in the regime where FLASH accelerators operate.

Comparing to candidate physical substrates.

Each of the candidate substrates for M(t) discussed in Chapter 15—calcium signalling, ion channel gating, redox dynamics, bioelectric membrane dynamics—carries its own characteristic timescale, determined by well-established biophysics. The question is which, if any, naturally produces relaxation on the 10–100 ms scale.

The most direct calculation is for bioelectric membrane dynamics. A cell membrane behaves, to first approximation, as an RC circuit, with resistance R_m provided by ion channel leak conductance and capacitance C_m provided by the lipid bilayer itself. The relaxation timescale is simply:

$$\tau = R\_m \cdot C\_m$$

The specific capacitance of cell membranes is essentially constant across cell types and well-constrained experimentally: $C\_m \approx 1\ \mu F/cm^2$. Membrane resistance varies substantially with cell type and physiological state: R_m ranges from approximately 10^3 Ω·cm² in electrically active tissues (cardiac muscle, neurons) to 10^5 Ω·cm² in more quiescent tissue. Substituting:

$$R\_m = 10^3\ \Omega\cdot\text{cm}^2 \rightarrow \tau = 1\ \text{ms}\ R\_m = 10^5\ \Omega\cdot\text{cm}^2 \rightarrow \tau = 100\ \text{ms}$$

The membrane RC timescale spans approximately 1–100 ms across the physiologically relevant range of tissue membrane resistance. This range is not chosen to fit the FLASH observation; it follows from a single textbook relation and two parameter values independently measured across decades of electrophysiology.

The convergence and what it means.

Two independent calculations give overlapping ranges:

From FLASH pulse-spacing phenomenology: $\tau\_M \approx 10 - 100$ ms

From membrane RC biophysics: $\tau = R\_m \cdot C\_m \approx 1 - 100$ ms

The overlap is approximately 10–100 ms. This is not a precise numerical match—both ranges are order-of-magnitude estimates. It is also not a uniqueness result: other biological substrates with fast dynamics (voltage-gated calcium channels, some rapid redox processes) can produce sub-second relaxation as well. What the convergence establishes is more modest: that *at least one* biological substrate—the bioelectric membrane dynamics invoked as the substrate of s_t in Chapter 10—naturally produces a decay timescale in the range the framework's FLASH prediction requires, without tuning of parameters and without invoking processes outside textbook membrane biophysics.

Seen this way, the numerical consistency is a sanity check rather than a proof. A framework that requires $\tau\_M \approx 10$–100 ms would be in difficulty if no known biological process produced relaxation in that range, or if the only candidates required specific fine-tuning to reach it. What the check shows is that the framework's requirement is satisfied by the specific substrate it proposes, using parameters the electrophysiology literature established independently. The agreement is between two numbers that were neither chosen nor tuned to match.

What this does and does not demonstrate.

What this check demonstrates: the framework's requirement on τ_M is not arbitrary, and the specific biological substrate it proposes—membrane RC dynamics—produces timescales in the required range using parameters independent of the radiotherapy context. The numbers meet.

What it does not demonstrate: that bioelectric dynamics are the substrate of M(t) in clinical tumours. That is a hypothesis the T2.1 pulse-spacing experiment, combined with T2.3 (direct oxygen dynamics measurement during FLASH delivery), is designed to test. A positive result on T2.1 with the predicted $\exp(-\gamma\ \Delta t)$ functional form and a fitted γ corresponding to τ_M in the 10–100 ms range would be consistent with the membrane RC interpretation. A positive result with τ_M outside this range would force the framework to identify a different candidate substrate from among those with compatible dynamics.

The check performed here is therefore a precondition for the experimental programme, not a substitute for it. The framework's fast-layer timescale and the most plausible candidate biological substrate agree at the order-of-magnitude level. That is the minimum a mechanistically grounded framework should be able to show before its predictions are tested in the laboratory.

SFRT as Spatial State Probings

Spatially Fractionated Radiotherapy deliberately delivers radiation in highly non-uniform patterns—grid or lattice arrangements that leave substantial tumor volumes receiving low or no dose in any given fraction. By the logic of spatial independence, this should be inferior to uniform irradiation: untreated regions should continue growing while treated regions respond. Yet SFRT has demonstrated effective and sometimes striking tumor control, particularly in bulky tumors that respond poorly to conventional approaches (Mohiuddin et al., 1999; Griffin et al., 2020). Irradiated regions influence non-irradiated ones. The response is not local. The tumor is behaving as a coupled system.

In the conventional framework, this requires invoking bystander effects, immune activation, and vascular changes as separate mechanisms—each contributing partially, none sufficient alone, and no framework integrating them into a coherent prediction.

In the informational state framework, SFRT is the spatial analog of FLASH. Just as FLASH drives the state along a temporal trajectory by modulating the timing of dose delivery, SFRT drives the state along a spatial trajectory by modulating the spatial distribution of dose. A spatially structured perturbation—high dose here, low dose there—does not produce locally contained responses. It propagates through the organizational coupling structure of the tumor, influencing the state of neighboring regions through the mechanisms that the Interaction Rule describes and that TCI detects.

The key variable is the tumor's spatial coupling strength—the degree to which perturbations in one region propagate through the informational state to influence adjacent regions. In a tumor with high TCI—strong organizational coupling—a spatially structured dose pattern will propagate extensively, producing non-local effects across the tumor. In a tumor with low TCI—fragmented dynamics, weak coupling—the same spatially structured dose pattern will produce primarily local effects, and the non-local coordination that makes SFRT effective will be absent.

This is the first place in the book where TCI becomes directly actionable rather than merely descriptive. TCI, measured from serial ADC imaging during MR-guided radiotherapy, predicts how SFRT will behave in a specific tumor. A high TCI is an indication that spatial fractionation will produce non-local effects—that the organizational coupling will propagate the perturbation across the tumor and engage the system-level response that makes SFRT effective. A low TCI suggests that spatial fractionation will produce primarily local effects—that the tumor's organizational fragmentation will limit propagation, and that a more spatially uniform approach may be more appropriate.

The spatial coupling structure is also the dimension of the informational state that SFRT most directly probes. A tumor's response to a spatially structured perturbation—whether the high-dose peaks produce effects that extend into the low-dose valleys, and how far—is a readout of the organizational coupling structure that generated those effects. The observation updates the belief state about the tumor's TCI and, more broadly, about which organizational configurations are consistent with the observed response pattern.

SFRT is not a niche technique for bulk tumors. It is a spatial probe of the informational state—a tool for perturbing the tumor's organizational coupling structure and observing how perturbations propagate. In the AIG-ART framework, it is deployed when TCI suggests strong coupling that spatial probing can exploit, and when the belief state about the tumor's organizational structure is broad enough that an informative spatial perturbation would substantially sharpen the estimate.

SBRT as Magnitude-Driven State Transition

Stereotactic Body Radiotherapy delivers high doses per fraction—five, ten, fifteen, twenty Gray—in a small number of treatments. Its clinical success is genuine and substantial, particularly for early-stage lung cancer and oligometastatic disease (Timmerman et al., 2010). But as Chapter 4 documented, its success coexists with a theoretical deficit: the LQ model breaks down at high doses per fraction, biological equivalence calculations become unstable, and outcome variability persists even when delivery is highly precise.

The informational state framework resolves this without requiring new mechanisms.

Large doses per fraction are large perturbations to the informational state. In a nonlinear dynamical system—which the tumor is, by the Nonlinearity Rule—large perturbations do not simply produce proportionally larger versions of what small perturbations produce. They can drive the system across bifurcations in state space, initiating qualitatively different trajectories from those that small perturbations initiate. The regime the system enters after crossing a threshold has different stability properties, different accessible configurations, different response characteristics. This is not a failure of the LQ model to accommodate high-dose biology. It is a consequence of the system's nonlinear state space producing qualitatively different dynamics above and below the threshold.

The threshold itself is a property of the tumor's informational state—not a fixed biological parameter but a characteristic of the current organizational configuration. Two tumors with the same genomic profile, the same histology, the same measured molecular characteristics can have different thresholds for regime transition, because they are in different informational states. This is the variability that dose alone cannot explain, and that the State Rule predicts: response depends on s_t, and s_t varies between tumors in ways that current measurements do not capture.

The variability in SBRT outcomes, seen from this perspective, is not noise to be reduced by better delivery precision. It is a signal—a reflection of the distribution of informational states across the patient population, each state determining the threshold for regime transition and therefore the trajectory initiated by a given high-dose fraction. Two patients receiving identical SBRT regimens are not receiving identical perturbations to their informational states. They are receiving the same physical dose, but the state-dependent effect of that dose—which regime it pushes the system into, which trajectory it initiates—depends on the state the treatment encounters.

In the AIG-ART framework, SBRT is a magnitude probe. It tests the boundary of the system's current dynamical regime—probing whether the state is in a configuration where a large perturbation will drive a favorable state transition (tumor control, immune activation, vascular disruption leading to indirect tumor cell death) or an unfavorable one (resistance-inducing reorganization, accelerated adaptive dynamics). The observation of how the tumor responds to a high-dose fraction—whether it enters a rapidly responsive trajectory or begins adaptive reorganization—updates the belief state about the system's regime boundaries and informs whether subsequent fractions should continue at high dose or shift strategy.

A Unified Interpretation

The three anomalies, viewed through the informational state framework, reveal a single picture rather than three separate puzzles. FLASH, SFRT, and SBRT each probe a different dimension of the informational state along a different axis of intervention—temporal dynamics, spatial coupling structure, and nonlinear regime boundaries respectively. Each produces observations that are more informative about the informational state than uniform conventional fractionation, precisely because each perturbs the system in a dimension that conventional fractionation holds constant. They are not merely clinical techniques in the AIG-ART framework. They are the primary experimental instruments through which the hidden state is made partially visible. They are the probes.

From Anomaly to Instrument

The practical consequence of this reinterpretation is a shift in how these modalities are thought about and deployed.

In the conventional framework, each modality is a treatment technique—something to be applied when clinically indicated, according to protocols developed from dose-response data, selected based on tumor size, stage, and location. FLASH is experimental. SFRT is for bulky tumors. SBRT is for oligometastatic disease and early-stage primaries. The selection criteria are largely anatomical and clinical, not organizational.

In the AIG-ART framework, the selection of modality is a decision about which dimension of the informational state to probe and perturb at this moment, given the current belief state and the expected informational value of each probe. A tumor with high TCI and a broad belief distribution about its spatial coupling structure calls for a spatial probe—SFRT. A tumor with a well-characterized coupling structure but uncertain temporal sensitivity calls for a temporal probe—FLASH. A tumor whose regime boundaries are poorly estimated calls for a magnitude probe—SBRT at a dose carefully chosen to approach but not blindly cross the estimated threshold. Chapter 16 develops how the machine combines these probes within a single fraction.

The Generalized Radiobiological Model

Having reinterpreted the anomalies through the informational state framework, it is now possible to state the generalized radiobiological model that subsumes them all.

The classical LQ model assum7es response is a fixed function of dose: $R = \alpha D + \beta D^2$. The parameters α and β are constants—intrinsic properties of the tissue, invariant across delivery conditions. This model is recovered as a special case when the informational state is constant and interaction terms are negligible—the conditions under which conventional fractionation at moderate doses is delivered, and under which the LQ model provides useful approximations.

The generalized model replaces fixed parameters with state-dependent ones:

$$R = \alpha(s_t)D + \beta(s_t)D^2 + I(s_t, \dot{T}, S, P)$$

where $\alpha(s_t)$ and $\beta(s_t)$ are the state-dependent radiosensitivity parameters—functions of the organizational state rather than constants—and $I(s_t, \dot{T}, S, P)$ is the interaction term capturing effects arising from temporal delivery structure $\dot{T}$, spatial fractionation pattern S, and particle type P—delivery dimensions whose biological consequences depend on the informational state and cannot be reduced to a simple dose-response relationship. The LQ model is recovered when s_t is constant and I vanishes. The full mathematical specification of this model, including the functional forms of $\alpha(s_t)$, $\beta(s_t)$, and $I(s_t, \dot{T}, S, P)$, and the state evolution equation that governs how s_t changes between and during fractions, is developed in Appendix A.

One caveat is necessary. The state-dependent parameters $\alpha(s_t)$ and $\beta(s_t)$ are theoretically derived—their functional forms follow from the M-ROD dynamics and the TCI coupling framework developed in Appendix A. They have not been empirically fitted to tumour data. No clinical measurement of $\alpha(s_t)$ or $\beta(s_t)$ has yet been made in any patient or tumour model. The generalised model is a theoretical architecture awaiting experimental characterisation, not a calibrated clinical tool.

The state-dependent forms $\alpha(s_t)$, $\beta(s_t)$, and $I(s_t, \dot{T}, S, P)$ are the framework's formal commitment to the Constraint Rule of Chapter 11. In conventional radiobiology, α and β are fixed tissue constants: component-level properties the system carries independently of any organizational context. Here they are functions of the state. Two tissues with identical molecular machinery but different organizational configurations will have different α and β, because the state modulates component-level radiosensitivity multiplicatively through the $M(s_t)$ and $TCI(s_t)$ terms developed in Appendix A. This is what operationalizing top-down causation looks like in the formal architecture: state-level variables setting the terms under which component-level biology responds, rather than the component-level biology determining the state. The same commitment extends to inference, through the belief state $b_t(s)$ developed in Chapter 13, and to decision-making, through the expected free energy action selector developed in Chapter 15. Whether a fully hierarchical formalism—in which slow layers strictly constrain fast ones—is required is an open question, addressed partially in the layer-coupling equations of Appendix A.2.2.

What this model makes explicit is that every parameter radiobiology treats as a constant is, in reality, a function of the informational state. Radiosensitivity is not a fixed tissue property. It is the current value of a state-dependent function—varying with the organizational configuration of the tumor, shifting as the state evolves under treatment, and determining the trajectory of response in a way that no measurement of α and β at baseline can predict.

This is the theoretical unification that the book has been building toward. FLASH, SFRT, and SBRT are not anomalies requiring special explanations. They are regimes in which the state-dependence of radiosensitivity becomes undeniable—regimes where the approximation of treating α and β as constants breaks down completely, and where the state-dependent generalized model is required. Conventional fractionation is the regime where the approximation holds well enough to be clinically useful. It is a special case of the more general theory, not the theory itself.

A note on the scope of the free energy framing

FEP enters this framework at two levels of commitment, and the asymmetry is deliberate. For resistance and the AIG-ART treatment architecture, FEP is load-bearing: the tumour's adaptive response to repeated treatment is a slow, cumulative, convergent process with the structural signature of inference, where weaker framings genuinely lose explanatory content. For the three anomalies—FLASH, SFRT, SBRT—the framework stays at the level of nonlinear dynamical systems: state, coupling, regime, bifurcation. FEP is compatible with these readings and provides their eventual dynamical backbone, but is not the primary explanatory engine here, because the anomalies are acute perturbations shaped as much by biophysics—membrane timescales, vascular thresholds, spatial coupling—as by inference. The division is principled rather than incomplete: FEP where inference is the dominant mode of organization, dynamical systems where biophysical dynamics carry the explanatory load, and an explicit bridge between them wherever the two must meet.

Toward the Control Framework

The anomalies have been reinterpreted. The generalized model has been stated. The three probing modalities have been placed in their correct positions as instruments for state inference rather than merely treatment techniques.

What remains is to build the complete AIG-ART control architecture—the system that takes the belief state, selects actions according to expected free energy minimization, delivers treatment across multiple modality dimensions simultaneously, observes the response, updates the belief, and selects the next action. This is the framework that uses everything built in Parts II and III to guide tumor control in the way that the informational state framework implies it must be guided: not through fixed protocol optimization, but through adaptive, inference-driven control of a partially observable dynamical system.

Chapter 15 develops the decision-making framework. Chapter 16 assembles the complete AIG-ART system.

PART IV

The AIG-ART Framework

Parts I through III made an argument. Part IV follows it to its conclusion.

The machine described in Chapter 16 does not exist in its complete form. The clinical scenarios of Chapter 17 are set in 2036 for a reason—they are not predictions but implications. If the framework is correct, this is the direction it points. If the experiments of Appendix D confirm the framework's core claims, this is what becomes possible. The chapters that follow should be read in that spirit: not as a proposal for what will be built, but as a precise answer to the question of what the informational state framework logically demands of a treatment system.

The decision-making architecture of Chapter 15 is grounded in established mathematics—POMDP theory, active inference, evolutionary game theory. The machine of Chapter 16 is grounded in existing hardware—MR-linac, proton pencil beam scanning, photoacoustic imaging—combined in ways that do not yet exist clinically but require no new physics. The clinical scenarios of Chapter 17 require only that the framework's predictions hold and that the engineering follows.

Read Part IV as the framework thinking out loud about its own consequences. That is what it is.

CHAPTER

15

Decision-Making Under Uncertainty: The Control Problem

What has not yet been built is the decision architecture—the machinery that takes the belief state and produces a treatment decision. That is what this chapter constructs.

It has one central argument: radiotherapy, understood correctly, is not a planning problem. It is a control problem. The difference is not semantic. It determines how treatment is designed, how it adapts, how it handles uncertainty, and how it responds to the tumor's own adaptive dynamics. Getting the problem formulation right is the prerequisite for everything that follows.

From Planning to Control

Conventional radiotherapy is organized around a plan. Before treatment begins, imaging is acquired, a target volume is delineated, dose constraints are specified, and an optimization algorithm finds the beam parameters that best satisfies those constraints. The plan is then executed—typically over five weeks—with modifications only when anatomical changes force a replan. The system is treated as known at the outset, static between replans, and predictable throughout.

This is planning. It is the appropriate problem formulation for a system that is fully observable, stationary, and deterministic. The tumor's informational state is none of these things.

The informational state is partially observable—the plan is optimized against a projection of the state, not the state itself. It is dynamic—the state evolves continuously under treatment, adaptation, and the tumor's own internal dynamics. And it is path-dependent—the state that exists at fraction ten depends on the actions taken at fractions one through nine, in ways that no baseline plan can fully anticipate.

Planning under these conditions produces a systematic error. The plan is optimal for the state assumed at baseline. But the actual state at any given fraction may differ substantially from the assumed state—because the baseline measurement was a projection, because the state has evolved since baseline, and because the treatment itself has been driving the state along a trajectory that the plan did not model. The plan continues executing against a tumor that has moved away from the model it was built on.

Control is the correct alternative. A control problem does not require knowing the state in advance. It requires a policy—a mapping from belief states to actions—that specifies what to do given whatever state estimate is currently available, however uncertain. The policy is not fixed at the outset. It is applied at each decision point, given the current belief, and the belief is updated between decision points as new observations arrive. The treatment adapts continuously—not to geometric changes in anatomy, but to inferred changes in the tumor's organizational state.

This is the conceptual shift that AIG-ART requires. Not better planning. A different kind of problem entirely.

The Full Action Space

Before the control problem can be solved, the action space must be defined precisely. What can the AIG-ART machine actually control?

In conventional radiotherapy, the primary control variable is dose magnitude D—the amount of radiation delivered per fraction, distributed spatially according to the optimized plan. Everything else is largely fixed by machine capability and protocol. AIG-ART extends this to a multi-dimensional action vector:

$$a_t = (D_t, \dot{T}_t, S_t, P_t, \pi_t, B_t)$$

Each component is a degree of freedom that the machine controls independently and simultaneously.

D_t is dose magnitude—how much radiation is delivered. The conventional variable, now understood as one dimension of a richer control space rather than the primary quantity to be optimized.

$\dot{T}_t$ is temporal structure—the dose rate, pulse spacing, duty cycle, and irradiation sequence. This is the FLASH dimension. It controls how the state variable M(t) in the M-ROD model evolves during delivery—specifically, how quickly the protective state activates, how long it persists, and how sensitively it depends on the temporal pattern of pulses.

S_t is spatial fractionation pattern—the distribution of dose across the tumor volume, including the grid and lattice patterns of SFRT as special cases. This controls how the spatial coupling structure of the state—the TCI dimension—is engaged. A spatially structured perturbation in a strongly coupled tumor propagates through the organizational state and engages system-level responses that uniform delivery cannot produce.

P_t is particle type—photon, electron, or proton. Each particle interacts with tissue differently, depositing energy with different spatial precision and different biological effectiveness per unit physical dose. The choice of particle at any moment determines which dimension of the informational state is being perturbed most strongly: protons for deep, spatially precise state transitions at the Bragg peak; electrons for FLASH delivery at ultra-high dose rates with sharp depth cutoff; photons for broad organizational perturbation across the full treatment volume.

π_t is the sequencing policy—the order and timing of individual delivery segments within a fraction. Which spot is delivered when, with what inter-spot interval, in what spatial sequence. This controls the interaction between delivery segments through the state: segments delivered in close temporal succession interact through the accumulated state, amplifying biological effect. Segments separated by multiples of the state decay timescale $1/\gamma$ interact minimally, reducing cumulative state accumulation in normal tissue. Temporal decoherence—the deliberate spacing of delivery segments to control interaction—is a direct implementation of the M-ROD decay dynamics as a clinical control parameter.

B_t is bioelectric field modulation—the application of low-intensity external electric fields between or during radiation pulses to manipulate the tumor's gap junctional connectivity and thereby its spatial coupling strength. This is the most speculative of the six dimensions: unlike dose magnitude, temporal structure, spatial pattern, particle type, and sequencing—each of which has experimental grounding—bioelectric field modulation is a prediction of the framework, not a validated control parameter. The biological basis is established in Chapter 10: gap junctional conductance is dynamically regulated by membrane potential, and external electric fields can shift this conductance in ways that increase or decrease the tumor's organizational coupling. Whether that shift can be achieved with sufficient tissue selectivity in vivo remains to be demonstrated. Appendix D prediction specifies the experiment required.

Conventional radiotherapy occupies a single point in this space—a specific D_t, with $\dot{T}_t$ fixed at conventional rates, S_t fixed at uniform distribution, P_t fixed by machine type, π_t determined by delivery efficiency rather than biological strategy, and B_t absent entirely. AIG-ART explores the full space, selecting the combination that minimizes expected free energy given the current belief state.

The Low-Dose Probing Pulse

Before the therapeutic action is executed, the AIG-ART machine performs a preliminary observation that is entirely new to radiotherapy practice: a low-dose probing pulse.

The probing pulse delivers a sub-therapeutic dose—far below the threshold of any clinically significant biological effect—to the tumor volume. Its purpose is not treatment. Its purpose is information. The pulse perturbs the system minimally and the tumor's response to that perturbation is recorded across all available sensing modalities simultaneously: the MR diffusion response, the PET signal change, the EIT impedance shift, and—through the Cherenkov emission or photoacoustic signal—the oxygen dynamics O(t) during the pulse.

Each of these responses is a state-discriminating observation. Different organizational states produce different responses to the same probing pulse. A tumor with high spatial coupling (high TCI) produces a response that propagates beyond the directly irradiated volume. A tumor with activated M(t) produces a response consistent with reduced radiosensitivity. A tumor in a resistant organizational configuration produces a response that diverges from the prediction of the current best-estimate state.

The inference engine processes these responses simultaneously and updates the belief state $b_t(s)$ before the therapeutic pulse is delivered. The update sharpens the belief—eliminating organizational configurations inconsistent with the observed response and increasing the credibility of configurations consistent with it. The therapeutic pulse that follows is then selected based on a more precise belief state than was available from imaging alone.

This is active inference at its most direct clinical expression: probing the system before acting on it, using the probe response to reduce uncertainty, and committing to the therapeutic action with better information than any pre-treatment imaging could provide. The additional dose from the probing pulse is negligible—subtherapeutic by design, contributing far less to the cumulative dose budget than the uncertainty in dose calculation that conventional planning already accepts. To be precise: a 0.1–0.3 Gy probing pulse represents less than 0.5% of a standard 60 Gy course prescription—smaller than the inter-fraction dose variation that adaptive radiotherapy already tolerates routinely.

The POMDP Policy: From Belief to Action

With the belief state $b_t(s)$ updated by the probing pulse response, the policy selects the therapeutic action. The policy π^* maps belief states to actions by minimizing expected free energy G(a)—the criterion established in Chapter 13.

In practical terms, this works as follows. For each candidate action in the action space, the policy simulates its expected effect across the distribution of possible states represented in the current belief. For each possible state s in the belief, the simulation predicts: what will the response be if the tumor is in state s and action a is applied? What will the imaging response look like? How will the state evolve? What will the next belief state be?

These predictions are aggregated across the full belief distribution, weighted by the probability of each state. The aggregation produces, for each candidate action, three quantities:

The expected extrinsic value—the expected therapeutic benefit, weighted across possible states. This is the treatment objective: drive the state toward configurations associated with tumor control, weighted by how likely each state is.

The expected epistemic value—the expected reduction in belief uncertainty that the action will produce. Actions that generate responses that strongly discriminate between plausible states score highly here—they tell the inference engine more about which state the tumor is actually in, enabling better decisions in subsequent fractions.

The expected complexity cost—the penalty for actions that deviate substantially from what the current belief predicts as normal. When the belief distribution is broad and many states are plausible, this cost is high—aggressive actions that would be catastrophic in some plausible states are penalized even if they would be optimal in others. This is clinical caution engineered directly into the decision criterion.

The policy selects the action that minimizes the sum of these three components—maximizing therapeutic effect and information gain while paying the appropriate cost for uncertainty. The full mathematical derivation of this optimization, including the specific functional forms of the three components and the algorithm for computing the optimal action, is given in Appendix A.

The Exploitation-Exploration Trajectory

The balance between these three components changes systematically as treatment progresses and the belief state evolves. This produces a characteristic trajectory in the policy—from exploration-dominant early treatment to exploitation-dominant late treatment—that is not imposed externally but emerges naturally from expected free energy minimization.

At the beginning of treatment, the belief state is broad. Many organizational configurations are plausible, because little has been observed about this specific tumor's state dynamics. The epistemic value of informative actions is high. The complexity cost is also high—aggressive actions are penalized because some plausible states would respond very poorly to them. The policy therefore favors probing-dominant actions: treatment fractions designed to generate maximally informative responses, at doses and in delivery configurations that sacrifice some immediate therapeutic efficiency in exchange for large uncertainty reduction.

Consider what this looks like clinically. Fraction one might deliver a spatially structured dose—an SFRT-like pattern—not primarily for its therapeutic effect but because the spatial response pattern reveals the tumor's TCI with high precision. Fraction two might switch to FLASH delivery—not primarily for normal tissue sparing but because the response to ultra-high dose rate reveals where M(t) activates and how quickly, constraining the oxygen memory component of the state. Fraction three might deliver a conventionally fractionated proton dose to test the system's response at the Bragg peak depth, revealing regime boundary information. After three fractions the belief state is far sharper than it would have been after three identical conventional fractions, and the policy is now far better positioned to exploit that belief.

As fractions accumulate and the belief sharpens, epistemic value decreases, complexity cost decreases, and extrinsic value dominates—the policy transitions toward aggressive therapeutic exploitation of the now well-characterized state. The machine does not need to be told when to shift from probing to exploiting. It shifts automatically as the belief evolves.

The Game-Theoretic Layer: Playing Against an Adaptive Opponent

Everything described so far treats the tumor as a dynamical system whose state is to be inferred and guided—appropriate for the fast timescale of organizational state evolution within and between fractions. At the slower timescale of evolutionary dynamics—the selection and expansion of clonal populations over a multi-week treatment—the tumor is also an adaptive opponent, responding to the treatment policy through Darwinian selection rather than deterministic state evolution.

This introduces a second layer to the control problem. The fast POMDP loop operates at the fraction and sub-fraction timescale. The slow game-theoretic loop—evolutionary state assessment, policy update, Stackelberg strategy recalibration—operates at the timescale of days to weeks.

The tumor's evolutionary dynamics are modeled as a strategic response to the treatment policy: given a fixed, predictable policy, the evolutionary dynamics will find configurations that survive it, and resistance will emerge (Gatenby et al., 2009; Zhang et al., 2017). The clinician's policy must therefore be designed not only to be optimal against the current state, but to be robust against the tumor's anticipated evolutionary response. The Stackelberg game structure formalizes this: the clinician moves first, selecting a policy; the tumor responds, its evolutionary dynamics adapting over subsequent fractions; the clinician must anticipate that response when selecting the policy, choosing not the policy that is optimal against the current state but the policy that remains effective even after the tumor has had the opportunity to adapt.

The Stackelberg game structure as a framework for managing evolving cancer systems has been independently developed and formalised by Stein et al. (2023) and Salvioli et al. (2024). The specific application here—using ctDNA-guided belief state updating to recalibrate the Stackelberg policy in real time across treatment fractions—extends that framework into the inference architecture of AIG-ART.

The adaptive therapy framework of Gatenby and colleagues established that a calibrated, non-maximum-dose policy guided by tumour burden monitoring can delay resistance by maintaining competitive suppression of sensitive clones—a clinical result that directly validates the game-theoretic logic of the slow loop (Gatenby et al., 2009; Zhang et al., 2017). What the AIG-ART architecture adds is the fast loop: an inference process operating at the pulse and fraction timescale, tracking the tumour's full organisational state across all four components rather than a single scalar observable such as PSA, and selecting actions across a six-dimensional delivery space that the adaptive therapy framework did not have access to. The slow loop inherits from Gatenby. The fast loop is new. The theoretical unification—the recognition that the evolutionary game and the radiobiological anomalies of FLASH, SFRT, and SBRT are all expressions of the same hidden organisational state—is what this book contributes beyond what either framework achieved alone.

The Stackelberg equilibrium is non-stationary by necessity. A fixed, repeating policy is a learnable signal: the tumor's evolutionary dynamics will converge on it given sufficient time and selection pressure. A machine with six control dimensions can present a policy that varies across temporal structure, spatial pattern, particle type, sequencing, and bioelectric modulation simultaneously—non-stationary in so many dimensions that evolutionary adaptation to any individual dimension leaves the others available for further variation.

The slow-loop inference—ctDNA monitoring between fractions, tracking which clonal populations are being depleted and which are persisting—feeds directly into the game-theoretic layer. As ctDNA reveals which organizational configurations are surviving, the Stackelberg policy updates to apply pressure through different control dimensions. The tumor's evolutionary dynamics and the clinician's policy co-evolve—each responding to the other—in a game whose outcome depends on which inference process is faster and more accurate.

The Evolutionary Trap

The most powerful clinical expression of the game-theoretic layer is the evolutionary trap—a specific policy design that exploits the tumor's competitive ecology to prevent resistance rather than simply delaying it.

The classical resistance failure mode is competitive release: treatment eliminates sensitive configurations, removing their competitive suppression of resistant ones, and resistant configurations expand into the vacated niche. Maximum dose kills sensitive configurations most efficiently—and therefore most efficiently releases the resistant ones (Gatenby et al., 2009).

The evolutionary trap inverts this logic. Rather than maximizing immediate cell killing, the policy maintains sensitive configurations alive at a controlled level—delivering a dose sufficient to prevent their expansion but insufficient to eliminate them—precisely because those sensitive configurations are suppressing the resistant ones. The sensitive population is kept as a competitive tool. Its presence prevents the resistant population from expanding. The tumor is held in a controlled equilibrium—not cured, but controlled.

Implementing this requires knowing where in the tumor sensitive and resistant configurations are spatially located—because the differential dosing must be spatially matched to the distribution of configurations. This is where the belief state and TCI connect to the evolutionary strategy. High-TCI regions indicate strong organizational coupling—regions where sensitive and resistant configurations are sharing organizational information through the bioelectric field and gap junctional connectivity. In these regions, the competitive suppression is most active. Disrupting the coupling—either through overdosing or through bioelectric field perturbation that reduces TCI—releases the resistant configurations. The policy must maintain the coupling in these regions at precisely the level that keeps competitive suppression operative.

This is the AIG-ART evolutionary strategy stated precisely: not maximum dose to maximum kill, but calibrated dose to maximum control, informed continuously by the belief state and ctDNA evolutionary monitoring, and designed to maintain the competitive ecology that prevents resistance from emerging rather than waiting for resistance to emerge and then attempting to overcome it.

The Therapeutic Window, Redefined

The therapeutic window—the gap between tumor control probability and normal tissue complication probability—is conventionally treated as a fixed biological ratio, determined by the intrinsic properties of tumor and normal tissue and only marginally modifiable by technical improvements in dose conformality.

The AIG-ART framework dissolves this fixity. The therapeutic window is a dynamic quantity—one that the treatment policy actively widens by exploiting the differential informational state between tumor and normal tissue across all six control dimensions simultaneously.

Each control dimension contributes a specific widening mechanism. Dose magnitude, optimized against the state-dependent generalized radiobiological model, selects the dose that maximally separates tumor state transition probability from normal tissue state transition probability. Temporal structure exploits the differential M(t) activation dynamics between tumor tissue—with disrupted organizational coherence—and normal tissue—with intact bioelectric connectivity—to achieve FLASH-mediated normal tissue protection selectively. Spatial pattern exploits the TCI differential between strongly coupled tumor and less coupled normal tissue to propagate organizational perturbations preferentially through the tumor. Particle type uses the Bragg peak to concentrate high-LET state transitions at the tumor depth while sparing normal tissue along the beam path. Sequencing policy uses temporal decoherence to reduce interaction-driven normal tissue damage while maintaining tumor interaction amplification. And bioelectric field modulation—when validated—could widen the window further by actively reducing normal tissue TCI while maintaining or enhancing tumor TCI.

These mechanisms are synergistic through the informational state—not additive, but superadditive. The total widening is greater than the sum of its parts because the control dimensions are coupled through the shared informational state framework. Chapter 16 assembles the machine that realizes this in practice.

The Framework at a Glance: Timescales, Substrates, and What s_t Adds

Before turning to how the machine works, it is worth stating plainly, in one place, how the framework's components relate to each other across timescales and what each contributes to the description of tumour behaviour under radiotherapy. A reader who has followed the argument this far will have encountered these distinctions in various chapters; this section assembles them.

Radiotherapy spans timescales from microseconds to weeks, and different physical and biological processes dominate in different regimes.

Microseconds to milliseconds. Radiation chemistry—radiolytic oxygen consumption, radical generation, peroxyl recombination, DNA damage induction. This regime is handled well by classical physicochemical models including ROD and its refinements. The informational state framework inherits these descriptions rather than replacing them; the oxygen dynamics O(t) in Appendix A are the same ROD equations radiobiology has used for decades. Chemistry at sub-millisecond scales is not where s_t contributes.

Tens of milliseconds to seconds. The fast layer of s_t, formalised as M(t) in the M-ROD model. This is where pulse-structure sensitivity, time-ordering dependence, and the FLASH threshold emerge—phenomena that chemistry alone cannot produce because memoryless models predict identical outcomes for irradiation schemes with matched total dose and average rate. M(t) is not a competing description of chemistry; it is the organizational memory coupled to chemistry, activated by dose-rate-dependent stress, and decaying on the characteristic timescale $1/\gamma$ that the T2.1 experiment is designed to measure. Its physical substrate is currently underdetermined—candidate implementations include redox-cooperative activation, calcium signaling, and ion channel state—and the framework's predictions distinguish among these without requiring commitment in advance.

Seconds to minutes biologically; days clinically. The spatial layer of s_t, denoted C(t). Bystander signalling, early immune activation, local vascular responses, and the organizational propagation of perturbations across tumour regions operate on seconds-to-minutes timescales biologically. But C(t) itself becomes clinically detectable only once serial diffusion-weighted MRI has accumulated enough fractions to resolve spatial structure—the Tumour Coupling Index developed in Chapter 12 first rises reliably above noise around fractions 3–5. Conventional radiobiology treats bystander and vascular effects as ad-hoc mechanisms added to explain specific anomalies; the informational state framework integrates them as consequences of s_t's spatial coupling structure. SFRT's non-local response is the clinical signature of this layer.

Minutes to hours—the intermediate biology. Between the fast regime of M(t) and the slow regimes below, there is real biology—DNA damage repair kinetics, cell cycle checkpoint response, early transcriptional activation, immune cell recruitment, vascular permeability changes. These are not a separate layer of s_t. They are distributed across the layers already named: the tail of M(t) relaxation for slowly-relaxing substrate components, the biological mechanisms that generate C(t), and the coupling between them. Radiobiology's established treatment of repair kinetics—the α and β parameters of the LQ model—is inherited here, generalised by the state-dependent forms $\alpha(s_t)$ and $\beta(s_t)$ developed in Chapter 14. Nothing is missing at this timescale; it is accounted for across the existing layers rather than by a dedicated one.

Days to weeks—the bioelectric layer B(t) and the epigenetic landscape. Here the framework draws on Levin's experimental work: bioelectric organizational states encode tissue-level memory that governs cellular behaviour, can be altered by physiological perturbation without genomic change, and persists across regeneration and turnover. Cancer involves disruption of this bioelectric coherence—a causal contribution to malignant behaviour, not merely its consequence. The informational state framework inherits Levin's substrate for its slow organizational regime, which operates on days to weeks and is tracked clinically by EIT from fractions 5–10. Epigenetic state transitions, documented without corresponding genomic changes, add a second slow layer coupled to the bioelectric one.

Weeks—the clonal architecture E(t). Selection under treatment pressure, competitive release of resistant subpopulations, and the tumour's adaptive response to a fixed treatment policy operate at this scale, tracked clinically by serial ctDNA from fraction 10 onward. This is where resistance-as-inference lives—the tumour's evolutionary dynamics functioning as a learning process against the clinician's strategy. Conventional models treat this regime statistically; the framework treats it dynamically.

Two clarifications follow from this layered picture.

First, the informational state is not composed of separate functional modules such as memory, signaling, or control. Rather, $s_t$is by construction a history-dependent, dynamical state, and each layer represents its realization at a particular timescale. The properties often described separately—memory, responsiveness, persistence—are intrinsic to the state at that scale, not additional components. Thus, $M(t)$, $C(t)$, $B(t)$, and $E(t)$ are not independent subsystems but scale-specific manifestations of the same underlying informational state. Each carries the system's history, constraints, and dynamics appropriate to its regime: fast organizational dynamics at the millisecond scale, spatially coupled propagation at intermediate scales, bioelectric patterning at longer times, and evolutionary adaptation at the longest scales. Figure 15.1 illustrates how these different time scales coupled with each other.

Second, the informational state does not compete with chemistry; it couples to it. Chemistry handles what happens below the resolution at which organizational states become dynamically relevant. M(t) takes oxygen dynamics as input; C(t) takes spatial damage distribution as input; B(t) responds to repeated treatment and adaptive signaling. The framework is not a replacement for physicochemical radiobiology—it is a multi-layer organizational description that sits above chemistry and captures what chemistry alone structurally cannot.

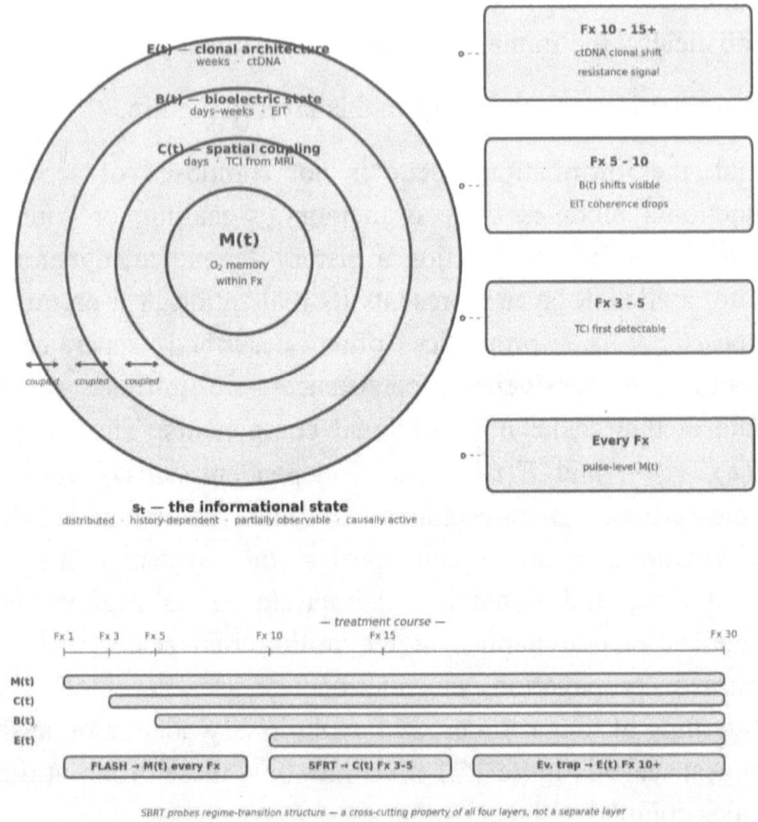

Figure 15.1. *Multiscale structure of the informational state s_t and its clinical observability. The informational state is organized as four coupled dynamical layers at differentimescales. M(t)—oxygen-memory activation—operates on tens of milliseconds to seconds within a fraction, probed by FLASH and measurable via Cherenkov and photoacoustic O_2 dynamics. C(t)—spatial coupling—is generated by biological mechanisms on seconds-to-minutes timescales but becomes clinically detectable as the Tumour Coupling Index from serial MRI only over days (fractions*

3–5), probed by SFRT. B(t)—the bioelectric organizational state grounded in Levin's experimental work (Chapter 10)—evolves over days to weeks and is tracked by EIT across fractions 5–10. E(t)—clonal architecture—evolves over weeks under selective pressure, tracked by serial ctDNA from fraction 10 onward, and is the target of the evolutionary trap. Sub-millisecond radiolysis drives M(t) via oxygen depletion but does not itself encode the history-dependent dynamics that define organizational memory; that memory requires cooperative, bounded dynamics with a characteristic decay timescale, which M(t) supplies. SBRT probes the nonlinear regime-transition structure of s_t*—a cross-cutting property of all four layers rather than a separate layer, which is why it does not appear as a row in the timeline.*

Limits of Inference and the Construction of the Machine

No inference system is immune to error. AIG-ART operates on incomplete, noisy observations of a partially observable tumour state, and its failures fall into two classes: inference failures, where the belief state misrepresents the underlying biology due to noise, model misspecification, or tracking lag; and delivery failures, where actions are suboptimal given the true state, particularly under conflicting signals or mistimed exploration. The system can be precisely wrong and will not recognise it. Its safeguards—sensing diversity, explicit uncertainty in the generative model, and conservative action under divergence—do not eliminate error; they bound its consequences.

These limits are structural, not correctable. The belief state therefore functions not only as an estimate of tumour state but as a signal of confidence, widening under contradiction and uncertainty and deferring to clinical judgement when resolution is not possible. The AIG-ART architecture is constructed with these failure modes in mind: an inference–action system designed to operate under partial observability rather than assume it away. The next chapter builds that machine explicitly.

CHAPTER

16

The Machine

The informational state framework demands sensing that goes beyond anatomy, inference that goes beyond planning, delivery that goes beyond dose, and adaptation that goes beyond geometric adjustment. The six rules, the POMDP policy, the two-timescale game-theoretic loop—none of these are computational abstractions. They are specifications. They describe, with mathematical precision, what a clinical system must be able to do. This chapter assembles that system.

It is not a radiotherapy machine with additional features. It is a categorically different kind of thing: a closed-loop biological control system that senses the tumor's hidden organizational state, infers its current configuration from incomplete observations, selects actions that simultaneously treat and probe, and updates its strategy continuously as the state evolves—at timescales ranging from milliseconds within a fraction to weeks across the treatment course. The machine that the informational state framework implies has never been built. This chapter describes what it would look like, what it would do, and why its capabilities are not additive but synergistic—emerging from the integration of sensing, inference, and delivery in ways that no individual component produces alone.

A New Kind of Thing

Begin with what is not new. MR-guided radiotherapy exists—the MR-linac combines real-time magnetic resonance imaging with photon delivery, enabling soft-tissue visualization during treatment. Proton pencil beam scanning exists—intensity-modulated proton therapy delivers dose with Bragg peak precision to complex target volumes. PET-guided radiotherapy exists—metabolic imaging informs dose painting and response assessment. Each of these represents a genuine advance. None of them, individually or together in their current form, constitutes what the informational state framework requires.

What is missing in each case is the same thing: the inference engine. Current MR-linac systems use real-time imaging for geometric guidance—ensuring the tumor is where the plan expects it to be. They do not use the imaging signal as a state observation that updates a probability distribution over organizational configurations and drives action selection. Current proton therapy systems optimize spot sequences for physical dose conformity. They do not reorder spots according to a biological state decay model calibrated in real time from the patient's tissue. Current PET guidance informs planning. It does not feed a continuous belief update running at the pulse timescale.

The AIG-ART machine is distinguished not by its components but by what connects them: a Bayesian inference engine that takes observations from all sensing modalities simultaneously, maintains a belief state $b_t(s)$ over possible organizational configurations, selects actions by minimizing expected free energy across the full six-dimensional delivery space, and updates continuously as the tumor's state evolves. The components serve the inference engine. The inference engine serves the framework. And the framework, as established across Parts II and III, is derived from the biology of the informational state itself.

The Physical Architecture

The machine is organized around a shared isocenter—the point in space where the tumor volume is positioned—and three concentric systems that surround it.

The innermost system is the delivery architecture: three particle delivery systems occupying the same treatment space, switchable within a fraction. The photon system provides broad, volumetric dose distribution through megavoltage photons—the standard modality for organizational perturbation across the full treatment volume. The electron system provides ultra-high dose rate capability through dedicated high-current electron acceleration—the FLASH modality, delivering dose at rates exceeding 40 Gy/s to exploit the M(t) differential between organized normal tissue and disorganized tumor tissue. The proton system provides pencil beam scanning through a compact proton gantry—the precision modality, placing Bragg peaks at specific depths with millimeter accuracy and enabling temporal decoherence of spot sequences through programmable inter-spot timing. A bioelectric field generator—four electrode arrays positioned around the treatment volume—delivers spatially structured low-intensity alternating electric fields between radiation pulses, modulating gap junctional conductance and thereby the tumor's TCI. This component is framework-derived and not yet experimentally validated; it is included here as the physical expression of the B_t control dimension, pending the confirmation described in Appendix D prediction T2.4. While the three particle systems are individually switchable within a fraction to match the inference engine's action selection, they are not mutually exclusive—the architecture supports concurrent delivery across multiple modalities when the optimal action requires it, such as proton pencil beam scanning combined with simultaneous bioelectric field modulation, or FLASH electron pulses interleaved with photon delivery to separate spatial targets within the same fraction. The action vector $a_t = (D_t, \dot{T}_t, S_t, P_t, \pi_t, B_t)$ is a simultaneous specification across all six dimensions—not a sequential menu—and the machine is designed to honour that specification in full when the belief state and clinical constraints permit.

The middle system is the sensing architecture: five modalities providing simultaneous, continuous observation of different dimensions of the informational state during and between delivery. The MR system—a 1.5 Tesla ring integrated coaxially with the delivery gantry—provides continuous diffusion-weighted imaging during treatment, generating the voxel-level ADC data from which TCI is computed in real time. The PET ring—integrated at the bore of the same magnet—provides simultaneous metabolic and functional imaging, tracking SUV changes across the tumor volume between pulse clusters. The EIT system—sixteen electrode arrays embedded in the patient positioning platform—measures tissue electrical impedance continuously throughout the fraction, providing a spatially resolved readout of the bioelectric organizational state that Chapter 10 established as a physical component of s_t. The photoacoustic system—external transducer arrays for accessible tumor volumes, with fiber-optic probes deployable endoscopically or interstitially for deep targets—measures oxygen dynamics O(t) in real time at and between pulses, providing direct readout of the fast physicochemical state variable in the M-ROD model. The Cherenkov emission system—a sensitive camera operating in the near-infrared, imaging the treatment surface during delivery—detects oxygen-sensitive luminescence during each radiation pulse for superficial and accessible tumor volumes, providing intrinsically co-registered O(t) measurement at the moment of dose delivery without additional dose or external light source.

These five sensing modalities do not operate in sequence. They operate concurrently, with co-acquisition logic matched to the timescale of each modality and the delivery structure. During active beam delivery: the MR system acquires diffusion-weighted images continuously—this is the defining capability of the MR-linac architecture; the EIT system measures impedance throughout, unaffected by the radiation field; and the Cherenkov camera captures oxygen-sensitive luminescence intrinsically co-registered to each pulse. Between pulse clusters: the PET ring acquires metabolic signal—beam-off periods are used precisely because scatter from active delivery degrades PET signal quality, making inter-pulse acquisition the correct strategy rather than a limitation; and the photoacoustic system captures O(t) recovery dynamics in the windows between pulses where the recovery curve is most informative. The inference engine receives all five data streams continuously and in parallel—not waiting for one modality to finish before processing the next. The belief state $b_t(s)$ is updated asynchronously as each new observation arrives from whichever modality generated it first. The machine is not a sequential pipeline. It is a parallel inference system operating at the timescale of the fastest modality—the Cherenkov camera and EIT, both operating within milliseconds of each pulse—while integrating the slower modalities as their observations arrive.

Between fractions, a sixth sensing dimension operates on the slower evolutionary timescale: an integrated microfluidic ctDNA analysis system processes a small blood draw collected at each fraction, providing clonal architecture information—which subpopulations are being eliminated, which are persisting, which are emerging—that feeds the game-theoretic slow loop.

The outermost system is the inference engine: a dedicated computational architecture running in real time alongside delivery. It maintains the generative model—the integrated M-ROD dynamics, TCI-coupling spatial model, bioelectric state evolution equations, and clonal competition dynamics—that connects states to observations and actions to state transitions. It runs the belief updater—a variational Bayesian algorithm that processes each new observation from every sensing modality and updates the probability distribution $b_t(s)$ over possible organizational configurations, operating at the pulse timescale. And it runs the action selector—the expected free energy minimizer that evaluates candidate actions from the six-dimensional delivery space and selects the combination that best balances extrinsic value, epistemic value, and complexity cost given the current belief.

The Two-Timescale Loop

The machine operates simultaneously on two timescales that feed the same belief state from different directions.

The fast loop runs within and between fractions, at the pulse-to-pulse timescale of milliseconds to seconds. It begins with a low-dose probing pulse—a sub-therapeutic delivery, typically 0.1 to 0.3 Gray, designed not for therapeutic effect but for maximal informational gain. The probing pulse perturbs the system minimally while generating simultaneous observations across all five sensing modalities: the MR diffusion response, the PET metabolic signal, the EIT impedance shift, the photoacoustic or Cherenkov O(t) signal. These responses are state-discriminating—different organizational configurations produce different responses to the same probing pulse, and the inference engine uses the response to sharpen the belief state before the therapeutic pulse is committed. The therapeutic pulse is then selected by the action selector from the full six-dimensional space, delivered, and its response observed. The belief is updated again. The next probing pulse is calibrated based on the updated belief. The loop runs continuously throughout the fraction: probe, observe, update, act, observe, update, probe.

The slow loop runs between fractions, at the fraction-to-fraction timescale of days to weeks. It takes as inputs the ctDNA clonal fractions from the inter-fraction liquid biopsy, the TCI trend computed from serial MR imaging across fractions, the SUV and mean ADC trajectories, and the cumulative OAR dose tracking. From these inputs the slow loop updates the evolutionary state estimate—which clonal configurations are currently dominant, how rapidly the clonal landscape is shifting, whether the evolutionary dynamics are consistent with the current Stackelberg policy or whether the policy needs recalibration. The fast loop and slow loop feed the same belief state $b_t(s)$—the fast loop updating the within-fraction organizational dynamics, the slow loop updating the between-fraction evolutionary dynamics. Together they provide the inference engine with the richest currently achievable partial observation of the tumor's informational state across all its timescales. Figure 16.1 illustrates these two time loops in a flow diagram.

The Inference Engine

The inference engine is not a treatment planning system that runs before the fraction and produces a fixed plan. It is a live computational process that runs during the fraction, updating continuously as observations arrive and selecting actions in real time.

Its core is the generative model—the integrated mathematical structure that connects states to observations and actions to state transitions. The generative model encodes the M-ROD oxygen dynamics, the TCI-coupling spatial propagation equations, the bioelectric state evolution model from Chapter 10, and the clonal competition dynamics of the game-theoretic layer. Given any organizational state and any action, the generative model predicts what the next state will be and what each sensing modality will observe.

The belief updater takes the current belief $b_t(s)$, receives a new observation o_t from the sensing architecture, and applies the Bayesian update equation through variational inference—approximating the true posterior over states with a tractable distribution that concentrates on organizational configurations consistent with the observation. The update runs at the pulse timescale. The full mathematical specification of the belief update algorithm, including the variational approximation and its convergence properties, is given in Appendix A.

The action selector takes the updated belief and evaluates candidate actions from the six-dimensional delivery space by computing expected free energy G(a) for each. The selected action minimizes G(a)—maximizing expected therapeutic effect and uncertainty reduction while paying the appropriate cost for clinical conservatism under uncertainty. Early in treatment, when the belief is broad, the action selector favors informative probing-dominant actions. As the belief sharpens across fractions, it transitions toward aggressive exploitation of the now-better-characterized state. This transition is not programmed—it is the natural output of the expected free energy optimization applied to an evolving belief.

The computational requirements are significant but not beyond current capability. Variational Bayesian inference over state spaces of clinically relevant dimensionality can be executed on modern GPU-accelerated hardware in milliseconds. The inference engine is an engineering challenge of the same kind as the challenges that produced the MR-linac and the proton pencil beam scanning system—

the next step in a progression that has, at each stage, required building new computational infrastructure to realize new clinical capability.

The Machine Running

What does the machine look like when it is operating?

The patient is positioned at the isocenter. The EIT electrodes are in contact. The Cherenkov camera is positioned. The photoacoustic probe—endoscopic for a deep pelvic target, external array for a breast tumor—is placed. A small blood draw has been processed overnight; the ctDNA clonal fractions are already loaded into the slow loop.

The inference engine activates. It loads the prior belief state from the previous fraction—the probability distribution over organizational configurations that accumulated from all prior observations and the overnight ctDNA analysis. It is not starting from scratch. It is continuing an inference process that has been running since the first treatment day.

The probing pulse is selected—the delivery configuration from the six-dimensional space that the action selector identifies as maximally informative given the current belief. A low-dose electron pulse at sub-therapeutic intensity, spatially structured to probe the coupling of the tumor's posterior margin. It is delivered in 200 milliseconds. The sensing architecture records the response across all five modalities—Cherenkov and EIT capturing within-pulse dynamics in real time, MR acquiring the diffusion response continuously, photoacoustic reading the O(t) recovery in the immediate post-pulse window, PET updating its metabolic estimate between pulse clusters. The belief updater processes the incoming streams asynchronously, integrating each modality's observation as it arrives. The full updated belief is available before the next heartbeat.

The action selector evaluates the therapeutic action space. Given the updated belief—which has just eliminated organizational configurations inconsistent with the probing pulse response—it selects the therapeutic pulse: proton pencil beam scanning with the temporally decoherent spot sequence calibrated to this patient's γ, spatial fractionation pattern matched to the TCI map, dose rate selected to exploit the confirmed M(t) differential. The therapeutic pulse is delivered. The Cherenkov camera tracks O(t) during delivery. If O(t) deviates from the model prediction, the inference engine flags an anomaly and adjusts the next pulse accordingly.

At the end of the fraction, the belief state $b_t(s)$ is archived. The ctDNA analysis from the current fraction's blood draw will be processed overnight and loaded into the slow loop before the next fraction begins. The Stackelberg policy for the next fraction is updated based on the day's evolutionary state estimate.

The machine does not rest between fractions. The slow loop continues processing. By the time the patient arrives for the next fraction, the inference engine already has a refined prior—and the game is already in progress.

Why the Capabilities Are Synergistic

The therapeutic window widening produced by the AIG-ART machine is not the sum of five independent improvements. It is a superadditive effect arising from the coupling of all capabilities through the shared informational state framework.

The FLASH-mediated normal tissue protection is more effective when the spatial fractionation pattern has pre-engaged the tumor's organizational coupling—because coupling propagates the protective state boundary more efficiently when the spatial structure is matched to the TCI map. The temporal decoherence that protects normal tissue creates precisely the inter-segment intervals during which the proton Bragg peak delivers its state transition to the tumor without interaction amplification in overlying tissue. The bioelectric field that enhances tumor TCI makes the SFRT spatial probe more informative to the inference engine, sharpening the belief state and enabling more precise dose selection, which reduces both underdosing and overdosing probability simultaneously. The probing pulse generates O(t) data that constrains the M-ROD state estimate, which improves the temporal sequencing policy, which improves the FLASH differential, which improves the NTCP prediction, which informs the reward function, which changes the action selected at the next fraction.

Each capability modifies the state in ways that alter what every other capability will produce. Remove any one and the remaining capabilities are weakened—not because they are individually dependent on it, but because the inference engine integrates them through a shared model, and a gap in the sensing or delivery architecture is a gap in the model's ability to track and manipulate the state.

This is what it means to build a machine from a framework rather than assembling a machine and then constructing a framework to describe it. Every component is present because the framework requires it. Every connection between components is made explicit by the framework. And the emergent capability—the closed-loop biological control system that plays an inference game against cancer—is the direct physical expression of the informational state theory of radiobiology developed across the preceding fifteen chapters.

Chapter 17 shows that machine in operation, facing five clinical opponents.

The Weight of Convergent Evidence

Before the clinical scenarios of Chapter 17 demonstrate the machine in operation, it is worth asking a question the reader is entitled to ask: how confident should we be, and in what specifically?

The argument of this book makes two distinct claims that carry different levels of evidential support, and they should be evaluated separately.

The first question: does a hidden internal state exist in tumours?

Here the argument rests on the mathematical argument that classical models are inadequate to the observational record. The identifiability theorem—proven by Koopmans (1949) and formalised for biological systems by Chis et al. (2011)

and Villaverde et al. (2016)—establishes that any system producing the observed pattern of failures must possess internal states not recoverable from observable outputs regardless of measurement precision. This is not probabilistic. It is a logical constraint on any model that tries to explain the observations without such states. The same inferential move has been made across five independent fields—macroeconomics (Lucas, 1976), control engineering (Kalman, 1960), neuroscience (Friston et al., 2017), pharmacokinetics (Jacquez and Perry, 1990), and ecology (Ludwig et al., 1978)—in each case forcing the recognition that aggregate observables do not uniquely determine internal configuration.

Independent experimental lines reinforce this structural argument. Gupta et al. (2011) and Marusyk et al. (2014) demonstrated phenotypic states interconvert independently of genomic change. Flavahan et al. (2017) demonstrated cancer cells exist in self-reinforcing history-dependent states causally active in determining treatment response. None of these studies were motivated by the present framework. Each arrives at the same structural conclusion from a different starting point: tumour behaviour is governed by configurations that are not reducible to the genomic or molecular measurements conventionally taken.

On this first question, the confidence is high. Not because any single experiment is decisive, but because the mathematical structure of identifiability forces the conclusion as soon as one accepts the observational record of FLASH, SFRT, and SBRT documented in Part I.

The second question: is that state informational and bioelectric in the specific sense this framework proposes?

Here the confidence is genuine but substantially lower. Davies (2019) has argued on physical grounds that living systems exhibiting goal-directed organisational maintenance are best understood as operating through causally active informational states; this book adopts that framing as a working position rather than a settled result. Pigozzi et al. (2025) demonstrated that gene regulatory networks can be trained to form associative memories in the Pavlovian sense, and that the trained state shows measurable changes in integrative causal emergence. Doan et al. (2026) showed associative conditioning in *Stentor coeruleus*, a single-celled organism without a nervous system. Levin's bioelectric work establishes experimentally that tissue-level organisational states can encode memory independently of genomic change, and can be deliberately altered through physiological means—but in model organisms (planaria, *Xenopus*), not in clinical tumours undergoing radiotherapy.

These lines of evidence are compatible with the framework and motivate it. They do not establish it. The specific claim that clinical tumours possess informational states that govern their response to radiotherapy, instantiated in bioelectric and related organisational substrates, remains a hypothesis. Appendix D specifies the experiments that would confirm or revise it.

What the two lines of argument together mean: there is strong reason to accept that some form of hidden state must exist in the systems radiotherapy treats. There is a coherent proposal—built on physical argument and experimental work in simpler systems—for what that state might be and how it might be detected and manipulated. The distance between the two is the distance between a structural argument and a clinical one, and it is honest to mark that distance clearly. The framework's job is not to close that distance by rhetoric. It is to specify the experiments that could close it empirically, and to commit to accept whatever those experiments return.

Transitioning to the final chapter of the book

This chapters described the machine in full—its delivery architecture, its sensing systems, its inference engine, and the synergistic logic that makes its capabilities more than the sum of their parts. What it did not show is the machine operating against real clinical problems.

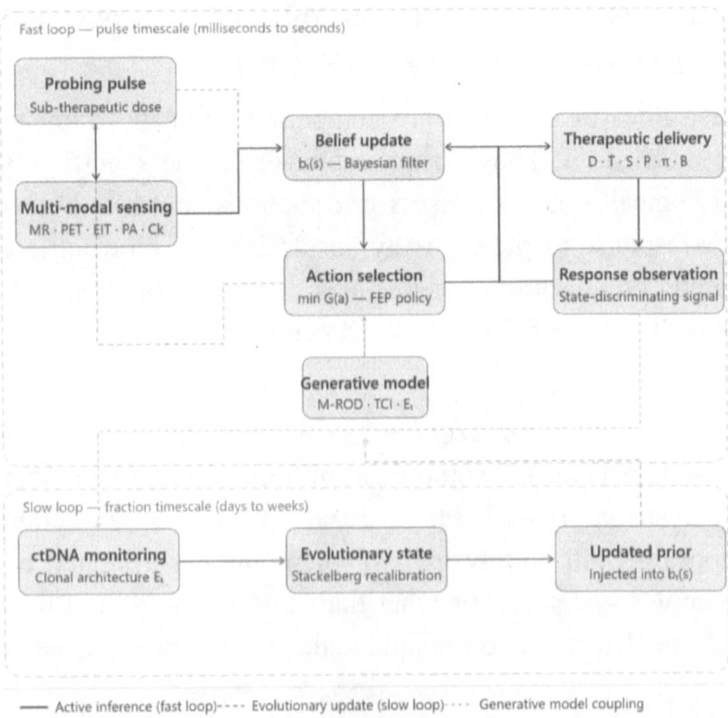

Figure 16.1. *Different components of the envisioned AIG-ART machine. The fast loop (solid arrows) operates at the pulse timescale: a sub-therapeutic probing pulse generates simultaneous observations across five sensing modalities; the inference engine updates the belief state $b_t(s)$ and selects the next six-dimensional therapeutic action via expected free energy minimisation G(a). The slow loop (dashed arrows) operates at the fraction timescale: ctDNA monitoring tracks clonal evolution; the Stackelberg policy recalibrates in response. Both loops share the same generative model.*

That is what the final chapter of this book – chapter 17 - does. Not as a prediction of what will happen, but as a precise answer to a question worth sitting with: if the framework is correct, what becomes possible that is not possible now? The five scenarios that follow are set in 2036 because that distance grants permission to think without the constraint of what currently exists. The biology is real. The mathematics is real. The clinical problems are ones you already face. Only the machine is imagined—and even that is imagined precisely, derived from specifications not wishes.

Table 16.1. Conventional radiotherapy versus AIG-ART: the essential differences

Dimension	Conventional radiotherapy	AIG-ART
Fundamental problem	Dose delivery: find the optimal spatial dose distribution for a static, fully characterised target.	State estimation and control: infer the tumour's hidden organisational state s-t and guide it toward desired configurations under uncertainty.

Tumour model	Static collection of clonogenic cells. Dose-response parameters α and β treated as fixed tissue constants.	Partially observable dynamical system with hidden state s-t. Parameters α(s-t) and β(s-t) are state-dependent and evolve continuously under treatment.
Role of uncertainty	Minimised or averaged away. Outcome variability is attributed to biological noise beyond the model's scope.	Explicitly represented as a probability distribution b-t(s) over possible organisational configurations. Managed through Bayesian inference, not suppressed.
Role of radiation	Damage-inducing agent. More dose is generally better. Delivery structure is secondary to total dose.	Perturbation and probe. Each fraction simultaneously treats the tumour and interrogates its hidden state. FLASH, SFRT, and SBRT probe distinct dimensions.
Resistance	Attributed to pre-existing resistant subclones or stochastic mutation. Managed after it becomes clinically apparent.	State transition: tumour evolves minimizing free energy. Intercepted proactively via signals like TCI reversal and ctDNA tracking.
Imaging role	Geometric verification: confirm tumour position. Imaging	State observation: imaging signals (ADC, SUV, etc.) update belief

	is a positioning tool.	distribution b-t(s).
Failure mode	Residual clonogenic cells cause recurrence.	State transition to resistant attractor; dynamic failure.
Objective function	Maximise TCP, minimise NTCP at prescribed dose.	Minimise expected free energy (tumour control + uncertainty reduction + complexity cost).
Evidential status	Clinically validated across decades. Parameters fitted to populations.	Theoretically grounded; clinical validation in progress.

CHAPTER

17

The Game: Five Clinical Scenarios

Imagine it is ten years from now—year 2036

The framework described in this book has been tested, refined, and partially validated. Some predictions held. Others required revision. The machine was built in stages—not all at once, and not exactly as described in the previous chapter, but close enough that the architecture would be recognisable. Radiation oncologists and medical physicists trained on it. Patients were treated with it.

What follows is a glimpse of what a morning in that clinic might look like—five patients, five treatment decisions, seen through the lens of a system that tracks the ghost rather than ignoring it. Nothing here has happened. But nothing here is impossible. The biology is real. The mathematics is real. The clinical problems are ones you already face every day.

Read it not as a claim about what has been achieved, but as an answer to a question worth sitting with: if the framework is right, what becomes possible that is not possible now?

Scenario 1—Locally Advanced Cervical Cancer: TCI-Guided SFRT with Bioelectric Sculpting

The patient.

A 44-year-old woman. FIGO IIB cervical cancer, a large tumour pressing against the posterior rectal wall—the kind of case where every beam path to the target passes through tissue you cannot afford to damage. Standard of care: chemoradiation to the pelvis, followed by brachytherapy boost. Yes we proudly continue using brachytherapy even in 2036—because its simple, targeted ionizing radiation just works!

What the machine sees that the conventional system does not.

The first two fractions are delivered as spatially structured probing pulses—not to maximise immediate cell kill, but to generate an informative response. The ADC signal propagates from the high-dose peaks into the adjacent untreated valleys. The TCI, computed from the voxel-level dynamics, is high. The tumour is strongly coupled—perturbations in one region propagate through the organisational network to its neighbours. Critically, the coupling is almost as strong at the posterior tumour-rectal interface as it is in the tumour core.

This is simultaneously the therapeutic opportunity and the danger. Organisational perturbations delivered to the tumour core will propagate toward the rectum through exactly the same coupling network that makes SFRT effective.

What the machine does differently.

Here the most speculative element of this vision enters—one that depends on the validation of Appendix D prediction T2.4, which has not yet been confirmed. On the assumption that bioelectric field modulation achieves sufficient tissue selectivity in vivo, the field generator is activated at the posterior field boundary between fractions—a low-intensity alternating field, targeted at reducing gap junctional conductance selectively at the tumour-rectal interface while preserving the coupling within the tumour core. Serial impedance monitoring tracks the effect fraction by fraction. The coupling differential widens. The spatial fractionation pattern concentrates its high-dose peaks in the anterior and lateral tumour bulk, where the maintained coupling can propagate the organisational disruption effectively. The posterior margin receives a lighter touch.

The small bowel, whose position shifts daily as bladder filling changes, is re-mapped at every fraction through the MR system. The delivery pattern updates accordingly. The rectum constraint is tracked in real time, not checked at planning and assumed stable.

What this means for the patient.

The therapeutic window is widened not by improving the geometry of the dose distribution—the physical plan is not dramatically different—but by managing the organisational biology of the interface. The tumour is disrupted through its own coupling network. The rectum is protected by actively reducing the coupling that would otherwise carry that disruption across the boundary. A conventional system delivers the same dose to the tumour-rectal interface as to the anterior tumour bulk, because it has no mechanism for distinguishing between them when they are separated by millimetres. This system creates that distinction in the biology, not the geometry.

Scenario 2—Left-Sided Breast Cancer: FLASH-Assisted Treatment with Cherenkov Cardiac Protection

The patient.

A 52-year-old woman. Left-sided triple-negative breast cancer, grade 3, post-lumpectomy. The tumour bed needs a boost. The left anterior descending artery runs behind the chest wall. Every Gray of mean heart dose carries a measurable increase in long-term coronary risk—a toxicity that will not declare itself for a decade, long after the oncologist has moved on and the patient has stopped thinking about radiation.

What the machine sees that the conventional system does not.

A low-dose FLASH probing pulse to the breast volume. The Cherenkov camera at the chest wall surface records the oxygen dynamics during the pulse. The myocardium, dense with connexin-43 gap junctions—among the most bioelectrically coherent tissue in the body—activates its protective state far more efficiently than the disorganised triple-negative tumour tissue. The differential is confirmed and quantified before the first therapeutic fraction is committed.

What the machine does differently.

Electron FLASH delivery to the whole breast, with the Cherenkov camera monitoring oxygen dynamics at the chest wall surface in real time during each pulse cluster. The temporal sequencing policy is governed by the M-ROD dynamics: pulse clusters are released when the cardiac protective state is fully engaged, held if oxygen recovery at the surface is incomplete. Delivery is cardiac-gated to systole, when the LAD is maximally displaced from the chest wall.

The axillary nodes are treated with proton pencil beam scanning. The Bragg peak sits at nodal depth; the sharp distal falloff protects the brachial plexus. Spots contributing overlapping dose to the plexus are temporally decoherent—spaced by multiples of the state decay timescale to prevent interaction-driven amplification of neural dose.

What this means for the patient.

The heart dose does not fall because the beams are aimed differently. It falls because the biology of the myocardium—its organisational coherence, its efficient activation of the protective state—is being exploited deliberately, in real time, in a way that the tumour tissue cannot match. The Cherenkov camera is not measuring dose. It is watching the biology respond and adjusting accordingly, within the fraction, while the patient is on the table.

The cardiac toxicity of left-sided breast radiotherapy accumulates silently over years. The system described here begins intercepting it from fraction one.

Scenario 3—Locally Advanced Rectal Cancer: Catching Resistance in the Act

The patient.

A 61-year-old man. T3N2 rectal adenocarcinoma, lower third, circumferential resection margin threatened posteriorly. Standard long-course chemoradiation. The surgical team is waiting. The question, as always, is whether the tumour will respond enough to make the operation feasible, and whether the response will last.

What the machine sees at fraction eleven.

The first ten fractions follow the expected trajectory. The tumour is shrinking. The diffusion signal is rising. The coupling index is falling—organisational disruption proceeding as planned. The ctDNA shows the dominant clonal population declining, a minor population slowly rising. Worth watching.

Fraction eleven. The diffusion signal continues to rise—good news by any conventional metric. But the coupling index reverses. It rises. And the ctDNA tells the same story from a different angle: the minor clone has become the majority.

The divergence is the key diagnostic. A system looking only at mean diffusion signal would report continued response and maintain the current plan for seventeen more fractions. What is actually happening is that cells are dying—hence the rising diffusion signal—but the survivors are reorganising into a more coupled, more coherent configuration. The rising coupling index is not a sign of tumour growth. It is a sign of tumour learning. The ghost is reorganising.

What the machine does differently.

The treatment strategy changes at fraction twelve—not because the tumour has declared clinical failure, but because the organisational state has signalled that the current strategy is producing adaptation rather than control.

The particle type switches from photon to proton. The spatial delivery pattern shifts to target the high-coupling subvolume identified by the spatial belief state—attempting to exploit the rising organisational coherence to drive disruption through the newly integrated resistant network before it fully stabilises. Simultaneously, the dose to subregions where the sensitive clone still has representation is moderated deliberately—not to spare those cells from charity, but to maintain them as competitive suppressors of the resistant clone. The evolutionary trap, set at fraction twelve.

By the final fractions, the coupling index has reversed again, falling back toward its pre-reversal level. The ctDNA shows the sensitive clone recovering. The response has been rescued.

What this means for the patient.

A conventional system, executing its pre-specified plan, would have delivered the same treatment for seventeen more fractions after the divergence signal—seventeen fractions of providing the resistant clone with a stationary, learnable treatment under no competitive pressure. The resistance that would have declared itself at surgical pathology, or as local recurrence six months later, was intercepted at the moment the organisational state made it visible. Two fractions before any conventional metric showed anything wrong.

Scenario 4—Oropharyngeal Cancer with Bilateral Nodes: Temporal Decoherence of IMPT Spots

The patient.

A 58-year-old man. HPV-positive base of tongue cancer, bilateral nodal disease. Proton therapy selected for superior organ-at-risk sparing. The plan requires hundreds of pencil beam spots across three beam angles. Many of those spots overlap in their contributions to the brainstem, the parotid glands, the spinal cord. In conventional raster scanning, these overlapping spots are delivered in rapid succession—effectively simultaneous from the perspective of the biological state.

What the machine measures before fraction one.

A single sub-therapeutic probing spot to the parotid region. The Cherenkov camera records the oxygen dynamics during the pulse. The M-ROD model fits the activation and decay dynamics to the signal and extracts the patient-specific decay time constant—not a population average from a reference dataset, but a measurement from this patient's parotid tissue on this day, reflecting whatever combination of hydration, prior dose, and bioelectric organisation currently characterises these glands.

The required decoherence interval for near-complete protective state recovery between overlapping parotid contributions follows directly from this measurement.

What the machine does differently.

The inference engine reorders all the spots from the raster scan to a temporally decoherent sequence. Brainstem-overlapping spots are distributed across the fraction with minimum decoherence intervals between consecutive brainstem contributions. Parotid-overlapping spots are similarly distributed. Spinal cord spots receive a more conservative margin—a serial structure, treated accordingly.

Simultaneously, spots within the primary tumour are deliberately clustered—delivered in rapid succession—to amplify interaction-driven biological effect through the tumour's organisational coupling. The same temporal parameter that protects the brainstem and parotids by decoherence amplifies tumour effect by deliberate coherence. One parameter. Opposite consequences at tumour and normal tissue. Derived from the same model, from a single probing pulse in the first minutes of fraction one.

The total fraction delivery time increases—this is the honest cost of the strategy, and it belongs on the table.

What this means for the patient.

Xerostomia is the toxicity that most consistently diminishes quality of life in long-term survivors of head and neck radiotherapy. It affects swallowing, sleep, speech, dental health, social function—often permanently. The parotid dose constraint exists because doses above a certain threshold reliably destroy salivary function. The temporal decoherence strategy does not change the physical dose to the parotid. The dose-volume histogram is essentially unchanged. What changes is the biological interaction of those doses through the organisational state—managed in real time, calibrated to this patient, updated each fraction as the state evolves.

Scenario 5—Oligometastatic Prostate Cancer: The Multi-Site Evolutionary Game

The patient.

A 68-year-old man. Gleason 4+4 prostate cancer with three synchronous bone metastases—lumbar spine, left iliac crest, right femoral neck. Combined with androgen deprivation therapy and a PD-1 checkpoint inhibitor initiated concurrently with radiation. The ctDNA at baseline shows three clonal populations: one androgen-sensitive and dominant, one intermediate, one carrying castration-resistant driver mutations and currently minor.

Four simultaneous radiation treatment problems. One shared evolutionary clock. And now, running alongside both, a fifth game: the immune system, newly unshackled by checkpoint blockade, learning which targets to pursue.

What the machine sees that changes everything.

Each lesion has its own informational state. The prostate primary is moderately coupled—the highest metabolic activity, the highest organisational coherence among the four sites. The spine lesion is similarly coupled. The iliac crest and femoral neck lesions are weakly coupled—fragmented dynamics, regions behaving more autonomously. Each lesion will respond differently to the same physical dose. Each lesion is part of the same clonal ecosystem, tracked through the shared ctDNA signal.

The machine is also tracking something the conventional system has never had a lens for: which lesion, irradiated in which way, is most likely to generate an immunogenic response capable of priming a systemic effect. Highly coupled tumour regions—where organisational coherence is intact—are the same regions where immune cell infiltration is most coordinated, where damage-associated signals propagate most efficiently through the tissue network, where the conditions for immunogenic cell death are most reliably met. The TCI is not only a measure of radiation response. In the presence of checkpoint blockade, it is also a partial map of immune opportunity.

The machine is playing four simultaneous radiation games, unified through a single evolutionary monitor—and a fifth game, played with the immune system as a partner rather than a bystander.

What the machine does differently.

The spine lesion is selected as the primary immune priming site. Its coupling index is moderate, its immune infiltration signature—read from the PET metabolic pattern and the EIT coherence—suggests an active rather than excluded immune microenvironment. The SBRT delivered here is not simply palliative. It is designed to generate maximal immunogenic cell death: spatially structured to engage the tumour's organisational coupling, temporally sequenced to avoid the immunosuppressive effects of continuous low-dose irradiation, timed to coincide with the peak T-cell expansion expected from the checkpoint inhibitor.

The prostate primary is treated with spatially structured delivery exploiting its moderate coupling—organisational perturbations propagated through the tumour network. The iliac crest and femoral neck lesions are treated as independent targets, their low coupling offering little to amplify.

After a handful of fractions, the ctDNA tells the machine something has shifted. The castration-resistant clone is rising—competitive release in progress as androgen deprivation eliminates the sensitive population. The slow loop raises an alert. The Stackelberg policy recalibrates. The dose to subregions where the sensitive clone still has representation is moderated deliberately—not from clinical timidity, but to maintain those cells as competitive suppressors of the resistant clone. The tumour is being treated differentially within itself, guided by what the evolutionary monitor reveals fraction by fraction.

Meanwhile, the ctDNA is being watched for a different signal: evidence of immune-mediated tumour reduction at a site that received no direct radiation. If the abscopal effect is emerging—if the immune response primed at the spine is beginning to act on the prostate or the iliac crest—the machine registers it in the belief state and adjusts the radiation strategy accordingly. A site where immunity is already working does not need the same radiation intensity as a site the immune system has not yet reached. The two treatments, radiation and immunotherapy, are no longer parallel tracks. They are coupled, each informing how the other is deployed.

What this means for the patient.

The abscopal effect has been documented, celebrated, and then frustratingly difficult to reproduce reliably. The reason it is unreliable is not that the biology is fragile. It is that we have been delivering radiation without any model of which lesion, irradiated in which way, at which moment relative to the immune cycle, is most likely to generate the systemic response we want.

The informational state framework offers the beginning of that model. The TCI identifies which tumour regions have the organisational coherence to generate coordinated immunogenic signals. The temporal sequencing policy controls the inflammatory character of the radiation—whether it produces the kind of cell death that activates immunity or the kind that suppresses it. The coupling between the radiation strategy and the ctDNA immune signal means the system knows, fraction by fraction, whether the intended immune priming is working and can adjust in response.

The prostate cancer story of the past two decades has been a story about clonal evolution outpacing treatment. In ten years, it may also become a story about learning to conduct three simultaneous strategies—evolutionary control, radiation delivery, and immune activation—as a single integrated campaign. The machine described here is what conducting that campaign might look like. This is not a cure. It is a different kind of intelligence brought to a problem that has defeated simpler approaches.

End Note

None of this has happened yet. The machine does not exist in this form. These patients are imagined.

But the problems they carry into the clinic are not imagined—you have seen versions of all five. The cervical tumour abutting the rectum. The rectal cancer that stops responding midway through. The prostate with three simultaneous metastatic sites pulling in different directions. These are Tuesday morning problems, familiar to every radiation oncologist who has practiced long enough.

What the framework offers is not a solution to those problems. Not yet. It offers a different way of seeing them—as state estimation problems, as inference games, as situations where the question is not only how much dose, but what is the system doing, and how do we stay ahead of it.

The experiments that would test whether this vision is achievable are specified in Appendix D. Some will confirm the framework. Some will force it to be revised. That is how it should be.

For now, the value of the thought experiment is simply this: you have seen what the ghost looks like when someone is finally looking for it. That image, once seen, is difficult to unsee.

Table 17.1—Five clinical scenarios mapped to primary state components, probe modalities and treatment modalities

Scenario	Primary state component	Probe modality	Treatment modality
1—Cervical (FIGO IIB)	B(t), C(t): Bioelectric coupling at tumour-rectal boundary	SFRT; Bioelectric field	Photon IMRT; Bioelectric field; Brachytherap y boost
2—Breast (Left-sided TNBC)	M(t): Differential O2-memory activation (myocardium vs tumour)	FLASH electron; Cherenkov	Electron FLASH; Proton IMPT
3—Rectal (T3N2)	C(t), E(t): TCI reversal + ctDNA clonal shift	Serial MRI; ctDNA	Photon IMRT → Proton IMPT
4—Oropharyngea l (HPV+ BOT)	M(t): Patient-specific decay constant γ	Proton probing pulse; Cherenkov	Proton IMPT
5—Prostate oligo (Gleason 4+4)	C(t), E(t), B(t): Shared ctDNA evolutionary clock	SBRT; ctDNA; PET + EIT	SBRT (spine, prostate, iliac + femur)

Epilogue
The Ghost, Revisited

The Preface of this book began with a confession. Radiotherapy, despite decades of technical refinement, despite the extraordinary precision of modern delivery systems, despite the biological knowledge accumulated in thousands of laboratories across the world, still fails in ways it cannot fully explain. Tumors that appear identical respond differently. Treatments that should work do not. Recurrence arrives not from untreated disease but from disease that was treated --- disease that learned, adapted, and survived precisely because of the treatment applied to it. Something was governing these outcomes that the framework being used to understand them could not see.

That something was given a name in Chapter 9. The informational state --- the distributed organizational configuration of the tumor that encodes its history, constrains its possible futures, and governs the behavior of its components through mechanisms that no molecular measurement can fully capture. The ghost in the cancer. Not supernatural. Not unknowable in principle. But hidden --- in the precise technical sense that a partially observable system is hidden: real, causally active, and accessible only through indirect inference from incomplete observations.

Fifteen chapters later, the framework has a body.

It has a mathematical structure — the state evolution equations of Appendix A, the TCI definition derived from the mean-signal invariance theorem, the POMDP architecture for inference under partial observability, the expected free energy decomposition for action selection. It has a candidate physical substrate, drawn from Levin's experimental work in planaria and *Xenopus*: the bioelectric field maintained across tissue through gap junctional coupling, encoding organizational memory without genomic change, alterable through physiological means. It has a coupling to the faster biology of radiation response through the M-ROD model — a memory-modulated extension of classical oxygen depletion whose decay timescale can in principle be measured in any patient with a single sub-therapeutic pulse. It has a candidate clinical instrument in TCI — computable from the voxel-level diffusion-weighted imaging data that MR-linac systems already acquire.

None of this has been proven in patients.

That sentence is the most important in the book, and it belongs here — not as a concession at the end of a triumphant argument but as the framework's actual epistemic position. The pattern of failures across FLASH, SFRT, and SBRT requires some form of hidden state by mathematical necessity. That requirement is structural and does not depend on the particular framework developed here. What this book has done beyond establishing the requirement is to propose a specific form for that state — informational, organizational, bioelectric — and to build the inference architecture that would act on it. The proposal is coherent. It draws on biological evidence that is direct and recent. It generates predictions specific enough to be tested. But it is a proposal, not a finding. The distance between "some hidden state must exist" and "the state has the specific form developed in this book" is the distance between a structural argument and an empirical one. The experiments in Appendix D are designed to close that distance — or to force the framework's revision when they return results that do not match what it predicts.

Three things are worth saying with particular clarity.

The first is that the argument for structural incompleteness of conventional radiobiology does not depend on this framework being correct. The identifiability problem is a mathematical result. A system with a distributed, history-dependent, partially observable internal state cannot be fully characterized by scalar imaging metrics, no matter how precisely those metrics are measured. This conclusion follows from the mathematics of dynamical systems and the biology of networked tissue organization. It does not require this book's specific proposal to be validated. It requires only that the observational record of Part I — FLASH, SFRT, SBRT failing the classical model along three different axes — is accepted. That conclusion stands whether or not the remainder of this framework survives its first contact with clinical data.

The second is that the biological evidence cited throughout the book is at different stages of establishment. The demonstrations of memory and learning in non-neural systems — Pigozzi et al. (2025) in gene regulatory networks, Doan et al. (2026) in *Stentor* — are direct experimental results and they are recent. The bioelectric work of Levin and colleagues in planaria and *Xenopus* is similarly direct, though in simpler model organisms. What has not been shown is that clinical tumours under radiotherapy possess organizational states of the kind these experiments establish elsewhere. That extrapolation is the specific claim this framework makes and the specific claim Appendix D commits to testing. It should not be confused with the evidence that made the extrapolation plausible in the first place.

The third is that the framework will almost certainly be wrong in specific predictions, even if its broad architecture is correct. The history of radiobiology is full of frameworks that were elegant, internally consistent, and ultimately wrong — or right in ways that turned out to be narrower than their proponents believed. The Linear Quadratic model itself, which this book has treated as an approximation to be generalized rather than a falsehood to be discarded, was once a contested theoretical construct that required decades of clinical experience to calibrate and qualify. The informational state framework may prove to be correct in its broad architecture and wrong in specific predictions. It may prove to be correct in some tumor types and inapplicable in others. It may generate clinical trials that confirm some of its mechanisms and falsify others, forcing revisions that the current version of the theory cannot anticipate. This is not a weakness. It is what a scientific theory is supposed to do.

The practical question is therefore not whether a hidden state exists in the systems radiotherapy treats — the mathematics forces this. The practical questions are whether the framework developed here correctly characterizes that state, whether the sensing modalities proposed can adequately observe it, whether the inference algorithms can track it with sufficient precision to guide treatment, and whether the clinical improvements illustrated in Chapter 17 actually materialize when the approach is tested prospectively. These are empirical questions. They have empirical answers. Those answers belong not to this book but to the experiments the book is trying to motivate.

The Preface of this book named a problem: that two patients, treated identically, can follow entirely different paths, and that the conventional framework of radiobiology has no account of why. That problem is real, and it has not gone away after fifteen chapters. What the framework offers is a specific proposal for what the conventional approach has been missing and a specific architecture for engaging it — tested in mathematics, grounded in biology from related systems, and committed to the experiments that would confirm or revise it. Whether the ghost in the cancer is real in the specific form this framework proposes, or real in some other form that better experiments will reveal, or whether the organizing image was misleading from the start and the problem is better described some other way entirely — these are things the next decade of work will determine. What the book argues, and what the next decade will test, is that the question is worth asking in this form. The rest belongs to the experiments and to the scientists and clinicians who will have the patience to run them.

Appendix A
Mathematical Development of the Informational State Framework

This appendix develops the complete mathematical structure of the Informational State framework for Adaptive Radiotherapy (AIG-ART). Every equation presented here is the formal expression of a concept introduced and motivated in the main text. The reader is assumed to have followed the conceptual argument of Parts I through IV. The purpose of this appendix is not to introduce new ideas but to make existing ones precise — to show that the intuitions built across seventeen chapters are not merely plausible but mathematically well-formed, and to provide the formal foundation from which the framework's predictions can be derived and tested.

The development proceeds in eleven sections, each building on the previous. Section A.1 introduces the generative model. Sections A.2 through A.4 derive the state evolution equations, M-ROD dynamics, and TCI framework. Section A.5 derives the observation models for each sensing modality. Sections A.6 through A.9 develop the inference and control architecture. Section A.10 formalizes the game-theoretic layer. Section A.11 derives the generalized TCP and NTCP models.

All notation is introduced at the point of first use and collected in Table A.1 at the end of this appendix for reference.

A.1 — The Generative Model

A generative model is a complete probabilistic specification of how observable data are produced from hidden causes. In the AIG-ART framework, the hidden cause is the tumor's informational state; the observable data are the outputs of the sensing architecture described in Chapter 16. The generative model has three components: the prior over initial states, the state transition distribution, and the observation distribution.

A.1.1 — The State Space

Let s denote a possible organizational configuration of the tumor. The informational state s_t at time t is an element of a state space $\mathcal{S}$ — the set of all organizational configurations the tumor system can occupy. $\mathcal{S}$ is a high-dimensional space whose axes correspond to the organizational dimensions established in Chapters 9 and 10: bioelectric field configuration, epigenetic landscape, gene regulatory network state, spatial phenotypic distribution, and clonal architecture.

In the computational implementation, $\mathcal{S}$ is approximated by a finite but large discrete space or by a continuous space with a tractable parametric structure. The choice of approximation determines the computational complexity of the inference algorithm and is addressed in Section A.6.

The tumor's informational state at time t is not a single point in $\mathcal{S}$ but a probability distribution over $\mathcal{S}$ — the belief state:

$$b_t(s) = p(s_t = s \mid o_{1:t}, a_{1:t-1})$$

where $o_{1:t}$ denotes the sequence of all observations from time 1 through t, and $a_{1:t-1}$ denotes the sequence of all actions from time 1 through $t-1$. The belief state is the posterior probability of each organizational configuration given everything that has been observed and done up to the current moment.

A.1.2 — The Prior

Before any observations are made — at the beginning of the first treatment fraction — the belief state is the prior distribution $p(s_0)$. In the AIG-ART framework, the prior is informed by baseline clinical measurements: tumor volume, baseline mean ADC, baseline SUV, baseline TCI, baseline EIT coherence, and baseline ctDNA clonal fractions. These measurements constrain which organizational configurations are plausible at treatment initiation.

Formally, the prior is constructed as:

$$p(s_0) \propto p(o_{\text{baseline}} \mid s_0) \cdot \tilde{p}(s_0)$$

where $\tilde{p}(s_0)$ is a weakly informative prior over the state space encoding general knowledge about tumor organizational states, and $p(o_{\text{baseline}} \mid s_0)$ is the likelihood of the baseline observations given each possible initial state.

A.1.3 — The State Transition Distribution

The History Rule (Rule 2, Chapter 11) states that the organizational state evolves as:

$$s_{t+1} = g(s_t, a_t, \omega_t)$$

where g is the state transition function, a_t is the action applied at time t, and ω_t is a stochastic process noise term representing biological variability and model uncertainty. In probabilistic form, this becomes the transition distribution:

$$p(s_{t+1} \mid s_t, a_t)$$

This distribution specifies the probability of transitioning to each possible next state, given the current state and the action taken.

A.1.4 — The Observation Distribution

Each sensing modality generates observations that are stochastic functions of the current state. Let $o_t = (o_t^{MR}, o_t^{PET}, o_t^{EIT}, o_t^{PA}, o_t^{ctDNA})$ denote the vector of observations from all five sensing modalities at time t. The observation distribution is:

$$p(o_t \mid s_t)$$

The complete generative model is the joint distribution:

$$p(s_{0:T}, o_{1:T} \mid a_{0:T-1}) = p(s_0) \cdot \prod_t p\,(s_{t+1} \mid s_t, a_t) \cdot p(o_t \mid s_t)$$

This factored form embodies the Markov assumption: the next state depends only on the current state and action, not on the full history. History-dependence is captured within the state itself through the History Rule, so the state transition is Markovian even though the observable tumor dynamics are not.

A.2 — The State Evolution Equation

The informational state s_t is a composite object with multiple components, each evolving on its own timescale and through its own dynamics.

A.2.1 — The State Vector

We decompose the informational state into four coupled components:

$$s_t = (M_t, C_t, B_t, E_t)$$

where:

$M_t \in [0,1]$ is the oxygen-memory activation state — the internal variable of the M-ROD model, representing the degree to which the system's temporal protective state has been activated by prior dose rate exposure. $M_t = 0$ represents the baseline unactivated state; $M_t = 1$ represents full activation. This component evolves on the fast timescale of tens of milliseconds to seconds during and between pulse deliveries, with characteristic decay rate γ (Section A.3.2) and $1/\gamma$ setting the temporal decoherence interval that determines pulse-structure sensitivity.

$C_t \in \mathbb{R}^{N \times N}$ is the spatial coupling matrix — a representation of the organizational coupling strength between spatial regions of the tumor, of which TCI is the scalar summary. The i,j entry of Ct represents the coupling strength between voxels i and j. The mechanisms that generate Ct — bystander signalling, early immune activation, vascular microenvironmental coupling — operate on timescales of seconds to minutes, but Ct itself accumulates and becomes clinically detectable as TCI from serial MRI over days (fractions 3–5; see Figure 15.1 and Appendix D prediction T3.1).

$B_t \in \mathbb{R}^N$ is the bioelectric state vector — the spatially resolved membrane potential distribution across the tumor volume. Following the experimental substrate established in Chapter 10 (Levin and colleagues), Bt evolves on the timescale of days to weeks, detectable via EIT across multiple fractions (fractions 5–10; see Figure 15.1 and Appendix D prediction T3.2).

$E_t \in \Delta^K$ is the clonal architecture vector — a probability simplex over K clonal populations, where each component E_t^k represents the fraction of the tumor's clonal burden attributable to subclone k. This satisfies $E_t^k \geq 0$ for all k and $\sum_k E_t^k = 1$. It evolves on the slow timescale of days to weeks under the selective pressure of treatment.

A.2.2 — Coupling Between Components

The four components are coupled through the biology established in Chapters 9 and 10.

The bioelectric state B_t determines the coupling matrix C_t:

$$C_t^{(i,j)} = \kappa\left(B_t^i, B_t^j\right) \cdot \exp(-\lambda \cdot d_{ij})$$

where $\kappa\left(B_t^i, B_t^j\right)$ is a coupling kernel that increases when the membrane potentials of voxels i and j are similar, d_{ij} is the Euclidean distance between voxels i and j, and $\lambda > 0$ is a spatial decay constant.

The clonal architecture E_t influences the bioelectric state B_t:

$$B_t^i = \sum_k E_t^{k(i)} \cdot \phi^k + \nu_i$$

where $E_t^{k(i)}$ is the fraction of voxel i attributable to clonal population k, ϕ^k is the characteristic membrane potential of clone k, and ν_i is a noise term representing spatial variability within each clonal population.

A.3 — The M-ROD Model: Formalizing Temporal State Dynamics

The M-ROD model describes the evolution of the oxygen-memory activation state M_t during and between radiation delivery.

A.3.1 — The Oxygen Depletion Equation

During radiation delivery, molecular oxygen in tissue is consumed through radiation-induced chemical reactions. Let $O(t) \in [0, O_0]$ denote the local oxygen concentration at time

t, where O_0 is the baseline concentration. The rate of oxygen depletion and subsequent re-oxygenation is governed by:

$$\frac{dO}{dt} = -k_D \cdot \dot{D}(t) \cdot O(t) + \frac{O_0 - O(t)}{\tau_O}$$

where $\dot{D}(t) \geq 0$ is the instantaneous dose rate (Gray per second), $k_D > 0$ is the oxygen depletion rate constant (Gray·second)$^{-1}$, and $\tau_O > 0$ is the oxygen recovery time constant (seconds).

The first term describes depletion: dose rate drives oxygen consumption proportional to both dose rate and current oxygen concentration. The second term describes re-oxygenation: vascular supply drives recovery toward baseline at rate $1/\tau_O$.

A.3.2 — The Activation Equation

The oxygen depletion $O_0 - O(t)$ drives activation of the internal protective state $M(t)$. The activation dynamics are:

$$\frac{dM}{dt} = \alpha_M \cdot \frac{[O_0 - O(t)]^n}{\theta^n + [O_0 - O(t)]^n} \cdot \big(1 - M(t)\big) + \beta_M \cdot M(t)\big(1 - M(t)\big) - \gamma \cdot M(t)$$

This equation has three terms:

Activation term: $\alpha_M \cdot \frac{[O_0 - O(t)]^n}{\theta^n + [O_0 - O(t)]^n} \cdot \big(1 - M(t)\big)$

The Hill function captures the cooperative, threshold-dependent nature of activation — sigmoidal in the oxygen depletion, rising steeply above threshold θ and saturating at 1.

The factor $(1 - M(t))$ ensures M cannot exceed 1. Parameters: $\alpha_M > 0$ (maximum activation rate, s^{-1}), $n > 1$ (Hill coefficient, dimensionless), $\theta > 0$ (half-activation oxygen depletion).

Positive feedback term: $\beta_M \cdot M(t)(1 - M(t))$

Once $M(t)$ begins to rise, activated components amplify further activation — a bistable switch mechanism. The logistic form $M(t)(1 - M(t))$ ensures feedback is maximal at intermediate values and vanishes at both extremes. Parameter: $\beta_M > 0$ (positive feedback rate, s^{-1}).

Decay term: $-\gamma \cdot M(t)$

In the absence of ongoing oxygen depletion, the activated protective state decays back toward $M = 0$ at rate γ. The reciprocal $1/\gamma$ defines the temporal decoherence interval for the spot sequencing policy of Chapter 15. Parameter: $\gamma > 0$ (decay rate constant, s^{-1}).

A.3.3 — Coupling to Spatial Organizational State

In a spatially extended tumor with coupling matrix C_t, the activation state $M(t)$ becomes a spatially resolved field $M(\mathbf{x}, t)$, governed by:

$$\frac{\partial M(\mathbf{x},t)}{\partial t} = \alpha_M \cdot F\big(O(\mathbf{x},t)\big) \cdot \big(1 - M(\mathbf{x},t)\big) + \beta_M \cdot M(\mathbf{x},t)\big(1 - M(\mathbf{x},t)\big) - \gamma \cdot M(\mathbf{x},t) + \delta \sum_{\mathbf{y}} C_t\,(\mathbf{x},\mathbf{y}) \cdot [M(\mathbf{y},t) - M(\mathbf{x},t)]$$

where $F\big(O(\mathbf{x},t)\big) = \frac{[O_0 - O(\mathbf{x},t)]^n}{\theta^n + [O_0 - O(\mathbf{x},t)]^n}$ is the Hill activation function at position **x**, and the spatial diffusion term $\delta \sum_{\mathbf{y}} C_t\,(\mathbf{x},\mathbf{y}) \cdot [M(\mathbf{y},t) - M(\mathbf{x},t)]$ couples the activation state at position **x** to neighboring positions **y** through the coupling matrix C_t. Parameter: $\delta > 0$ (spatial coupling coefficient, s^{-1}).

In normal tissue with high organizational coherence (high C_t values), this term propagates $M(\mathbf{x},t)$ rapidly across the tissue. In tumor tissue with disrupted coherence (low C_t values), propagation is limited. This differential propagation is the biological mechanism of the FLASH therapeutic window.

A.3.4 — The Radiosensitivity Function

The oxygen-memory activation state $M(\mathbf{x},t)$ modifies local radiosensitivity through:

$$\alpha_{\text{eff}}(\mathbf{x},t) = \alpha_0 \cdot [1 - \eta \cdot M(\mathbf{x},t)]$$

$$\beta_{\text{eff}}(\mathbf{x},t) = \beta_0 \cdot [1 - \eta \cdot M(\mathbf{x},t)]^2$$

where α_0 and β_0 are the baseline radiosensitivity parameters, and $\eta \in [0,1]$ is the maximum protection factor ($\eta = 1$ corresponding to complete radioprotection). When $M(\mathbf{x},t) = 0$, the effective parameters equal their baseline values —

recovering the standard LQ model. When $M(\mathbf{x}, t) = 1$, $\alpha_{\text{eff}} = \alpha_0(1 - \eta)$ and $\beta_{\text{eff}} = \beta_0(1 - \eta)^2$, giving the maximum protection effect.

A.4 — The TCI Framework: Formalizing the Interaction Rule

A.4.1 — The Spatial Tumor Model

Consider a tumor represented as N voxels, each with a state variable $x_i(t)$ representing the imaging-derived signal (e.g. ADC) at voxel i and time t. The dynamics of $x_i(t)$ are governed by:

$$\frac{dx_i}{dt} = f_i(x_i, s_t) + \sum_j C_t^{(i,j)} \cdot [x_j(t) - x_i(t)] + \varepsilon_i(t)$$

where $f_i(x_i, s_t)$ is the local dynamics function, $\sum_j C_t^{(i,j)} \cdot [x_j(t) - x_i(t)]$ is the coupling term (a discrete Laplacian), and $\varepsilon_i(t)$ is a zero-mean noise term with variance σ^2.

A.4.2 — The Mean Signal Invariance Theorem

Let $\bar{x}(t) = \frac{1}{N}\sum_i x_i(t)$ denote the mean signal across all voxels. Taking the mean of the voxel dynamics equation:

$$\frac{d\bar{x}}{dt} = \frac{1}{N}\sum_i f_i\,(x_i, s_t) + \frac{1}{N}\sum_i \sum_j C_t^{(i,j)} \cdot \left[x_j(t) - x_i(t)\right] + \frac{1}{N}\sum_i \varepsilon_i\,(t)$$

For a symmetric coupling matrix ($C_t^{(i,j)} = C_t^{(j,i)}$ for all i, j), swapping indices in the first inner sum gives:

$$\sum_i \sum_j C_t^{(i,j)} \cdot x_j(t) = \sum_j \sum_i C_t^{(j,i)} \cdot x_i(t) = \sum_i \sum_j C_t^{(i,j)} \cdot x_i(t)$$

Therefore the coupling term is exactly zero:

$$\frac{1}{N}\sum_i \sum_j C_t^{(i,j)} \cdot \left[x_j(t) - x_i(t)\right] = 0$$

The mean signal evolution reduces to:

$$\frac{d\bar{x}}{dt} = \frac{1}{N}\sum_i f_i\,(x_i, s_t) + \frac{1}{N}\sum_i \varepsilon_i\,(t)$$

This is independent of C_t. The coupling matrix — no matter how strong, no matter what structure it has — makes no contribution to the evolution of the mean tumor signal. Aggregate imaging metrics are mathematically blind to spatial coupling by pairwise symmetry.

A.4.3 — The TCI Definition

The Tumor Coupling Index is defined as the normalized reduction in prediction error achieved by incorporating spatial information:

$$\mathrm{TCI} = \frac{E_{\mathrm{ind}} - E_{\mathrm{spatial}}}{E_{\mathrm{ind}}}$$

where E_{ind} is the mean squared prediction error of the **independent model** — predicting each voxel's future signal using only that voxel's own history:

$$\hat{x}_i^{\mathrm{ind}}(t+1) = h_i\big(x_i(t), x_i(t-1), \ldots, x_i(t-p)\big)$$

$$E_{\mathrm{ind}} = \frac{1}{N}\sum_i \mathbb{E}\left[\left(x_i(t+1) - \hat{x}_i^{\mathrm{ind}}(t+1)\right)^2\right]$$

and E_{spatial} is the mean squared prediction error of the **spatial model** — predicting each voxel's future signal using both its own history and the current states of its spatial neighbors $\mathcal{N}(i)$:

$$\hat{x}_i^{\mathrm{spatial}}(t+1) = h_i^s\big(x_i(t), \ldots, x_i(t-p), \{x_j(t) : j \in \mathcal{N}(i)\}\big)$$

$$E_{\mathrm{spatial}} = \frac{1}{N}\sum_i \mathbb{E}\left[\left(x_i(t+1) - \hat{x}_i^{\mathrm{spatial}}(t+1)\right)^2\right]$$

The normalization ensures $\mathrm{TCI} \in [0,1)$. When $\mathrm{TCI} \approx 0$, the spatial model provides no predictive advantage — regions evolve independently. When $\mathrm{TCI} > 0$, knowing neighboring **regions genuinely improves prediction — organizational coupling is present and real.**

A.4.4 — Relationship Between TCI and the Coupling Matrix

In the linear case where $f_i(x_i, s_t) = -\lambda_i \cdot x_i$, the expected TCI can be expressed analytically in terms of the coupling matrix eigenstructure. Let μ_k and $\mathbf{v}_k$ denote the eigenvalues and eigenvectors of C_t. Then:

$$\mathbb{E}[\text{TCI}] = 1 - \frac{\sigma^2}{\sigma^2 + \sum_k \mu_k^2 \cdot \| \mathbf{P}_k \|^2}$$

where σ^2 is the noise variance and $\mathbf{P}_k$ is the projection of the voxel signal vector onto the kth eigenvector of C_t. Larger eigenvalues — corresponding to stronger coupling modes — contribute more to spatial predictability and therefore to TCI.

A.5 — The Observation Model

A.5.1 — MR Diffusion (ADC)

$$\text{ADC}_i = \text{ADC}_{\text{free}} \cdot (1 - f_{\text{cell}}) + \text{ADC}_{\text{cell}} \cdot f_{\text{cell}}$$

$$p(\text{ADC}_{i,t} \mid s_t) = \mathcal{N}(\text{ADC}_{i,t};\ \mu_{\text{ADC}}(s_t^i),\ \sigma_{\text{ADC}}^2)$$

where $\mu_{\text{ADC}}(s_t^i)$ is the expected ADC at voxel i given the local state, and σ_{ADC}^2 is the measurement noise variance.

A.5.2 — PET (SUV)

$$\text{SUV}_i = \rho \cdot \sum_k E_t^{k(i)} \cdot \phi_{\text{met}}^k + \xi_i$$

$$p(\text{SUV}_{i,t} \mid s_t) = \mathcal{N}(\text{SUV}_{i,t};\ \mu_{\text{SUV}}(s_t^i, E_t^i),\ \sigma_{\text{SUV}}^2)$$

where ρ is a scanner calibration constant, ϕ_{met}^{k} is the characteristic metabolic rate of clone k, and ξ_i is a noise term.

A.5.3 — EIT (Bioelectric State)

The impedance at frequency ω at spatial location **x**, modeled via the Cole-Cole equation:

$$Z(\mathbf{x}, \omega) = Z_\infty + \frac{Z_0 - Z_\infty}{1 + (i\omega\tau_{\text{EIT}})^{1-\alpha}}$$

where Z_0 is the zero-frequency impedance, Z_∞ is the infinite-frequency impedance, τ_{EIT} is the characteristic relaxation time, $\alpha \in [0,1]$ is a tissue heterogeneity parameter, and $i = \sqrt{-1}$.

$$p(\text{EIT}_t \mid s_t) = \prod_{\mathbf{x}} \mathcal{N}\left(Z(\mathbf{x}, \omega);\ \mu_Z(B_t^{\mathbf{x}}, C_t^{\mathbf{x}}),\ \sigma_{\text{EIT}}^2\right)$$

A.5.4 — Photoacoustic and Cherenkov Imaging (Oxygen Dynamics)

The photoacoustic signal:

$$\text{PA}(\mathbf{x}, t) = \Gamma \cdot \mu_a(\mathbf{x}, t) \cdot \Phi(\mathbf{x}, t)$$

$$p(\text{PA}_t \mid s_t) = \mathcal{N}\left(\text{PA}(\mathbf{x}, t);\ \mu_{\text{PA}}\left(O(\mathbf{x}, t)\right),\ \sigma_{\text{PA}}^2\right)$$

For Cherenkov-excited luminescence with an oxygen-sensitive phosphorescent probe (lifetime-based sensing):

$$\tau(\mathbf{x}, t) = \frac{\tau_0}{1 + k_q \cdot O(\mathbf{x}, t)}$$

$$O(\mathbf{x},t) = \frac{\tau_0/\tau(\mathbf{x},t) - 1}{k_q}$$

where τ_0 is the unquenched lifetime and k_q is the quenching rate constant of the probe.

A.5.5 — ctDNA (Clonal Architecture)

$$\psi^k = 1/2 \cdot E_t^k \cdot \rho_{\text{shed}}^k + \varepsilon^k$$

$$p(\text{ctDNA}_t \mid E_t) = \prod_k \mathcal{N}\left(\psi^k;\ 1/2 \cdot E_t^k \cdot \rho_{\text{shed}}^k,\ \sigma_{\text{ctDNA}}^2\right)$$

where ρ_{shed}^k is the shedding rate of clone k and ε^k is assay noise.

A.6 — The Belief State and Bayesian Update

Given the generative model of Section A.1 and the observation models of Section A.5, the belief state $b_t(s) = p(s_t = s \mid o_{1:t}, a_{1:t-1})$ is updated at each time step according to Bayes' theorem:

$$\begin{aligned} b_{t+1}(s') &= p(s_{t+1} = s' \mid o_{1:t+1}, a_{1:t}) \\ &\propto p(o_{t+1} \mid s_{t+1} = s') \\ &\cdot \int p(s_{t+1} = s' \mid s_t = s, a_t) \cdot b_t(s)\, ds \end{aligned}$$

This has two steps:

Prediction step — integrates the current belief forward through the state transition model:

$$\bar{b}_{t+1}(s') = \int p(s_{t+1} = s' \mid s_t = s, a_t) \cdot b_t(s)\, ds$$

Update step — incorporates the new observation:

$$b_{t+1}(s') = \frac{p(o_{t+1} \mid s_{t+1} = s') \cdot \bar{b}_{t+1}(s')}{p(o_{t+1} \mid o_{1:t}, a_{1:t})}$$

A.6.1 — The Variational Approximation

The exact Bayesian update is computationally intractable for high-dimensional state spaces. The AIG-ART inference engine uses variational Bayesian inference to approximate the true posterior with a tractable distribution $q(s)$ from a family $\mathcal{Q}$:

$$q^*(s) = \underset{q \in \mathcal{Q}}{\operatorname{argmin}} \ \mathrm{KL}[q(s) \ \| \ p(s \mid o_{1:t}, a_{1:t-1})]$$

where $\mathrm{KL}[q \parallel p] = \int q(s) \cdot \log\left[\frac{q(s)}{p(s|o_{1:t}, a_{1:t-1})}\right] ds$ is the Kullback-Leibler divergence.

The variational free energy $\mathcal{F}[q]$ is defined as:

$$\mathcal{F}[q] = \mathrm{KL}[q(s) \ \| \ p(s)] - \mathbb{E}_q[\log p(o_{1:t} \mid s, a_{1:t-1})]$$

The key identity connecting variational inference to the Free Energy Principle:

$$\mathrm{KL}[q(s) \ \| \ p(s \mid o_{1:t}, a_{1:t-1})] = \mathcal{F}[q] - \log p(o_{1:t} \mid a_{1:t-1})$$

Since $\log p(o_{1:t} \mid a_{1:t-1})$ is constant with respect to q, minimizing $\mathcal{F}[q]$ is equivalent to minimizing the KL divergence — finding the best approximation to the true posterior within $\mathcal{Q}$.

A.7 — The Generalized Radiobiological Model

A.7.1 — Deriving the LQ Model as a Special Case

The classical Linear Quadratic model describes the surviving fraction after dose D as:

$$\mathrm{SF} = \exp(-\alpha D - \beta D^2)$$

In the informational state framework, this is recovered as a special case when (1) the informational state s_t is constant throughout delivery, and (2) the interaction term $I(s_t, \pi) = 0$.

A.7.2 — The Generalized Model

The generalized radiobiological response function is:

$$R(D, s_t) = \alpha(s_t) \cdot D + \beta(s_t) \cdot D^2 + I(s_t, \dot{\mathrm{T}}, S, P)$$

where $\mathrm{SF} = \exp(-R)$. The state-dependent radiosensitivity parameters are:

$$\alpha(s_t) = \alpha_0 \cdot [1 - \eta \cdot M(s_t)] \cdot \left[1 + \zeta \cdot \left(1 - \mathrm{TCI}(s_t)\right)\right]$$

$$\beta(s_t) = \beta_0 \cdot [1 - \eta \cdot M(s_t)]^2 \cdot \left[1 + \zeta \cdot \left(1 - \mathrm{TCI}(s_t)\right)\right]$$

where $\eta \in [0,1]$ is the maximum $M(t)$-mediated radioprotection factor (Section A.3.4) and $\zeta > 0$ is the TCI-mediated radiosensitivity modulation factor.

The interaction term decomposes as:

$$I(s_t, \dot{T}, S, P) = I_{\text{temporal}}(s_t, \dot{T}) + I_{\text{spatial}}(s_t, S) + I_{\text{particle}}(s_t, P)$$

capturing effects from temporal sequencing, spatial structure, and particle type respectively that cannot be reduced to a simple dose-response relationship.

A.8 — The Free Energy Principle and Active Inference

A.8.1 — Variational Free Energy

The variational free energy decomposes as:

$$\mathcal{F}[q] = \underbrace{\text{KL}[q(s) \parallel p(s)]}_{\text{Complexity}} - \underbrace{\mathbb{E}_q[\log p(o \mid s)]}_{\text{Accuracy}}$$

Complexity measures how much the posterior belief $q(s)$ deviates from the prior $p(s)$. Accuracy measures how well the current belief explains the observations. Minimizing free energy finds the belief that best balances these competing pressures.

The connection to the evidence lower bound:

$$\log p(o) = -\mathcal{F}[q] + \text{KL}[q(s) \parallel p(s \mid o)]$$

Since $\text{KL}[q \parallel p(s|o)] \geq 0$, the variational free energy $\mathcal{F}[q]$ is an upper bound on $-\log p(o)$ — the surprise generated by the observations. Minimizing $\mathcal{F}[q]$ minimizes an upper bound on surprise.

A.8.2 — Expected Free Energy

The expected free energy $G(a)$ of action a is:

$$G(a) = \mathbb{E}_{q(s_t), p(s_{t+1}|s_t,a), p(o_{t+1}|s_{t+1})}[\log q(s_{t+1}) - \log p(o_{t+1}, s_{t+1})]$$

This decomposes into three terms:

$$G(a) = \underbrace{-\mathbb{E}[\log p(o_{t+1} \mid C)]}_{\text{Extrinsic value}} + \underbrace{\mathrm{KL}[q(s_{t+1} \mid a) \parallel p(s_{t+1})]}_{\text{Complexity cost}} \underbrace{- \mathbb{E}\big[\mathrm{KL}[q(s_{t+1} \mid o_{t+1}, a) \parallel q(s_{t+1} \mid a)]\big]}_{\text{Epistemic value}}$$

where C denotes the clinically desired (prior preferred) observations. The optimal action minimizes expected free energy:

$$a^* = \underset{a}{\operatorname{argmin}}\, G(a)$$

A.9 — The POMDP Formulation

The AIG-ART treatment optimization problem is a Partially Observable Markov Decision Process with the following components:

- **State space** $\mathcal{S}$: the space of informational state vectors $s = (M, C, B, E)$
- **Action space** $\mathcal{A}$: the six-dimensional delivery space $a_t = (D_t, \dot{T}_t, S_t, P_t, \pi_t, B_t)$
- **Transition model** $\mathcal{T}(s' \mid s, a) = p(s_{t+1} = s' \mid s_t = s, a_t = a)$

- **Observation model** $\mathcal{O}(o \mid s) = p(o_t = o \mid s_t = s)$
- **Reward function:**

$$R(s,a) = w_{\text{TCP}} \cdot \log\text{TCP}(s,a) + \sum_k w_k \cdot \log\left(1 - \text{NTCP}_k(s,a)\right) + w_{\text{QoL}} \cdot \text{QoL}(s,a)$$

- **Belief state** $b(s) = p(s \mid o_{1:t}, a_{1:t-1})$
- **Discount factor** $\gamma_{\text{disc}} \in [0,1]$

The optimal policy π^* minimizes expected cumulative free energy over the treatment course:

$$\pi^* = \underset{\pi}{\text{argmin}}\ \mathbb{E}\left[\sum_{t=0}^{T} \gamma_{\text{disc}}^t \cdot G(a_t) \mid \pi\right]$$

A.10 — The Game-Theoretic Layer: Stackelberg Dynamics

A.10.1 — The Replicator Equation

The evolution of the clonal architecture E_t under treatment is governed by the replicator dynamics:

$$\frac{dE_t^k}{dt} = E_t^k \cdot \left[f^k(E_t, a_t) - \bar{f}(E_t, a_t)\right]$$

where $f^k(E_t, a_t)$ is the fitness of clone k under action a_t, and $\bar{f}(E_t, a_t) = \sum_k E_t^k \cdot f^k(E_t, a_t)$ is the population mean fitness.

The fitness function:

$$f^k(E_t, a_t) = r^k - \delta^k(a_t) - \sum_j c^{kj} \cdot E_t^j$$

where $r^k > 0$ is the intrinsic growth rate of clone k, $\delta^k(a_t) \geq 0$ is the treatment-induced death rate, and $\sum_j c^{kj} \cdot E_t^j$ is the competitive suppression term with competition coefficients $c^{kj} > 0$.

A.10.2 — The Stackelberg Game

The clinician's objective is to maximize cumulative reward:

$$\max_{\pi} \sum_t R\,(s_t, a_t)$$

subject to the constraint that the clonal architecture evolves according to the replicator equation. The Stackelberg equilibrium policy is:

$$\pi_{\text{SE}} = \operatorname*{argmax}_{\pi} \sum_t R\left(s_t(\pi), a_t(\pi)\right)$$

where $s_t(\pi)$ denotes the state trajectory induced by policy π through the coupled dynamics of the belief update and the replicator equation.

The policy must vary faster than the timescale $\tau_{\text{evo}} = 1/\lambda_{\max}$ of the replicator dynamics, where $\lambda_{\max}$ is the largest eigenvalue of the Jacobian of the replicator equation at the current clonal architecture. The recalibration criterion:

$$\text{Recalibrate when:} \quad \left|\frac{dE_t^{\text{resistant}}}{dt}\right| > \varepsilon_{\text{thresh}}$$

A.11 — TCP and NTCP: The Generalized Models

A.11.1 — Generalized TCP

Under Poisson statistics, the tumor control probability is:

$$\mathrm{TCP} = \exp(-\lambda)$$

where $\lambda = N_0 \cdot \mathrm{SF}_{\mathrm{total}}$ and N_0 is the initial number of clonogenic cells. The surviving fraction after fraction t:

$$\mathrm{SF}_t = \exp\big(-R(D_t, s_t, \pi_t)\big)$$

The total surviving fraction after T fractions:

$$\mathrm{SF}_{\mathrm{total}} = \prod_{t=1}^{T} \mathrm{SF}_t = \exp\left(-\sum_{t=1}^{T} R\,(D_t, s_t, \pi_t)\right)$$

For a heterogeneous tumor with clonal architecture E_t:

$$\lambda = \sum_k N_0^k \cdot \exp\left(-\sum_t R^k\left(D_t, s_t^k, \pi_t\right)\right)$$

$$\mathrm{TCP} = \exp\left(-\sum_k N_0^k \cdot \exp\left(-\sum_t R^k\left(D_t, s_t^k, \pi_t\right)\right)\right)$$

The LQ-based TCP is recovered when all clones are identical and the state is constant with $M(s_0) = 0$ and $\mathrm{TCI}(s_0) = \mathrm{TCI}_0$.

A.11.2 — Generalized NTCP

The normal tissue complication probability using the Lyman-Kutcher-Burman framework, extended to incorporate state-dependent biological dose modification:

$$\mathrm{NTCP} = \Phi\left[\frac{D_{\mathrm{eff}}^{\mathrm{bio}} - \mathrm{TD}_{50}}{m \cdot \mathrm{TD}_{50}}\right]$$

where Φ is the normal cumulative distribution function, TD_{50} is the dose causing 50% complication probability, m is the normalized slope, and:

$$D_{\mathrm{eff}}^{\mathrm{bio}} = D_{\mathrm{eff}}^{\mathrm{phys}} \cdot [1 - \eta_{\mathrm{OAR}} \cdot M_{\mathrm{OAR}}]$$

where η_{OAR} is the maximum $M(t)$-mediated protection factor for the specific OAR and M_{OAR} is the mean $M(t)$ activation achieved in the OAR during delivery.

The predicted gain in uncomplicated control probability:

$$\Delta P^{+} = \mathrm{TCP} \times \left(1 - \mathrm{NTCP}_{\mathrm{primary}}\right) - \mathrm{TCP}_{\mathrm{LQ}} \times \left(1 - \mathrm{NTCP}_{\mathrm{primary}}^{\mathrm{LQ}}\right)$$

Table A.1 — Notation Reference

Symbol	**Definition**	**Units**	**First Introduced**
s_t	Informational state at time t	—	Section A.1.1
S	State space	—	Section A.1.1
$b_t(s)$	Belief state: $p(s_t = s \mid o_{1:t}, a_{1:t-1})$	Probability	Section A.1.1
o_t	Observation	Various	Section

	vector at time t		A.1.4
a_t	Action vector at time t: (D, $\dot{T}$, S, P, π, B)	Various	Section A.2
M_t	Oxygen-memory activation state	Dimensionless [0,1]	Section A.2.1
C_t	Spatial coupling matrix	Dimensionless	Section A.2.1
B_t	Bioelectric state vector	mV	Section A.2.1
E_t	Clonal architecture vector	Dimensionless $[0,1]^K$	Section A.2.1
O(x,t)	Oxygen concentration at position x, time t	mM	Section A.3.1
O_0	Baseline oxygen concentration	mM	Section A.3.1
$\dot{D}(t)$	Instantaneous dose rate	Gy/s	Section A.3.1
k_D	Oxygen depletion rate constant	$(Gy \cdot s)^{-1}$	Section A.3.1
τ_O	Oxygen recovery time constant	s	Section A.3.1
α_M	Maximum M(t) activation rate	s^{-1}	Section A.3.2
N	Hill coefficient for M(t) activation	Dimensionless	Section A.3.2
Θ	Half-activation oxygen depletion	mM	Section A.3.2
β_M	Positive feedback rate for M(t)	s^{-1}	Section A.3.2
Γ	M(t) decay rate constant	s^{-1} (or min^{-1})	Section A.3.2
Δ	Spatial coupling coefficient for	s^{-1}	Section A.3.3

	M(t)		
H	Maximum M(t)-mediated radioprotection factor	Dimensionless [0,1]	Section A.3.4
α_0, β_0	Baseline LQ radiosensitivity parameters	Gy^{-1}, Gy^{-2}	Section A.3.4
$\alpha(s_t)$, $\beta(s_t)$	State-dependent radiosensitivity parameters	Gy^{-1}, Gy^{-2}	Section A.7.2
Z	TCI-mediated radiosensitivity modulation	Dimensionless	Section A.7.2
TCI	Tumor Coupling Index	Dimensionless [0,1)	Section A.4.3
E_ind	Mean squared prediction error, independent model	(imaging units)^2	Section A.4.3
E_spatial	Mean squared prediction error, spatial model	(imaging units)^2	Section A.4.3
F[q]	Variational free energy	Nats	Section A.6.1
G(a)	Expected free energy of action a	Nats	Section A.8.2
E_t^k	Fraction of clone k in clonal architecture	Dimensionless [0,1]	Section A.2.1
f^k	Fitness of clone k	s^{-1}	Section A.10.1
r^k	Intrinsic growth rate of clone k	s^{-1}	Section A.10.1
δ^k	Treatment-induced	s^{-1}	Section

	death rate of clone k		A.10.1
c^{kj}	Competition coefficient between clones k and j	s^{-1}	Section A.10.1
TCP	Tumor control probability	Dimensionless [0,1]	Section A.11.1
NTCP	Normal tissue complication probability	Dimensionless [0,1]	Section A.11.2
TD_{50}	Dose causing 50% complication probability	Gy	Section A.11.2
m	LKB NTCP normalized slope parameter	Dimensionless	Section A.11.2
ΔP+	Gain in uncomplicated control probability	Dimensionless	Section A.11.2
N_0	Initial number of clonogenic cells	Dimensionless	Section A.11.1
SF	Surviving fraction	Dimensionless [0,1]	Section A.11.1
π*	Optimal POMDP policy	—	Section A.9
π_SE	Stackelberg equilibrium policy	—	Section A.10.2
γ_disc	POMDP discount factor	Dimensionless [0,1]	Section A.9

Appendix B
Computational Validation: Key Results

The mathematical framework developed in Appendix A makes specific, falsifiable predictions about how tumor systems should behave under controlled conditions. This appendix presents the key computational results from two preliminary studies — Vaitheeswaran (2026b) and Vaitheeswaran (2026a) — that test these predictions in simulation. Both studies are available in full at their respective preprint DOIs and are reproduced here under Creative Commons CC BY 4.0 license. These results constitute proof of principle, not clinical validation. They demonstrate that the model equations produce the behaviors the framework predicts — nothing more, nothing less.

B.1 — M-ROD: Temporal State Dynamics (Vaitheeswaran, 2026b)

The M-ROD model makes four predictions that distinguish it from classical ROD. Each was tested in simulation using the parameters of Table 1 of the preprint.

Prediction 1: LQ and ROD are recovered at conventional dose rates.

The State Rule requires that $\alpha(s_t)$ and $\beta(s_t)$ reduce to their baseline values when $M(t) \to 0$ — which the model predicts occurs when dose rate is far below the activation threshold D_c = 55 Gy/s. Figure B1 confirms this: at conventional dose rates (~0.01–0.1 Gy/s), M-ROD survival curves are indistinguishable from both ROD and LQ predictions. The internal state variable introduces no perturbation where the framework says it should not. At FLASH dose rates (~40–100 Gy/s), M-ROD diverges sharply from both, with substantially higher surviving fraction in normal tissue — the FLASH sparing effect emerges directly from the state dynamics.

Framework connection: Section A.7.1 — LQ recovery as special case; Section A.3.2 — M(t) activation threshold.

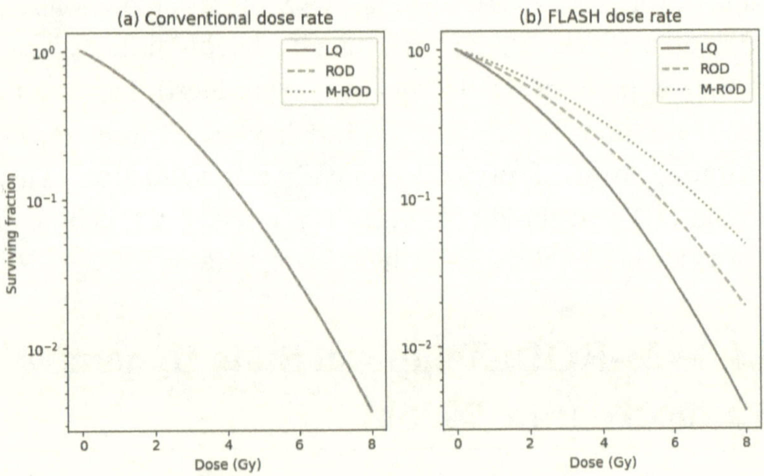

[Figure B1 — Survival as a function of dose: conventional vs FLASH dose rates. M-ROD reproduces LQ and ROD at low dose rates and diverges at FLASH rates. Source: Figure 1, Vaitheeswaran (2026b).]

Prediction 2: Dose-rate response is threshold-like, not smooth.

Classical ROD predicts a smooth, monotonically falling normal tissue response as dose rate increases. The M-ROD model predicts a sharp threshold-like onset followed by saturation — because the Hill function $f(\dot{D})$ creates a steep activation transition at D_c and the bounded nature of M enforces saturation. Figure B2 demonstrates this precisely: ROD produces a smooth curve across 0–200 Gy/s; M-ROD produces a sharp onset near D_c = 55 Gy/s and plateaus at high dose rates. This is the dose-rate signature of the FLASH effect.

Framework connection: Section A.3.2 — Hill function activation; nonlinear feedback term $\eta M^2(1\text{-}M)$*; Nonlinearity Rule (Rule 5).*

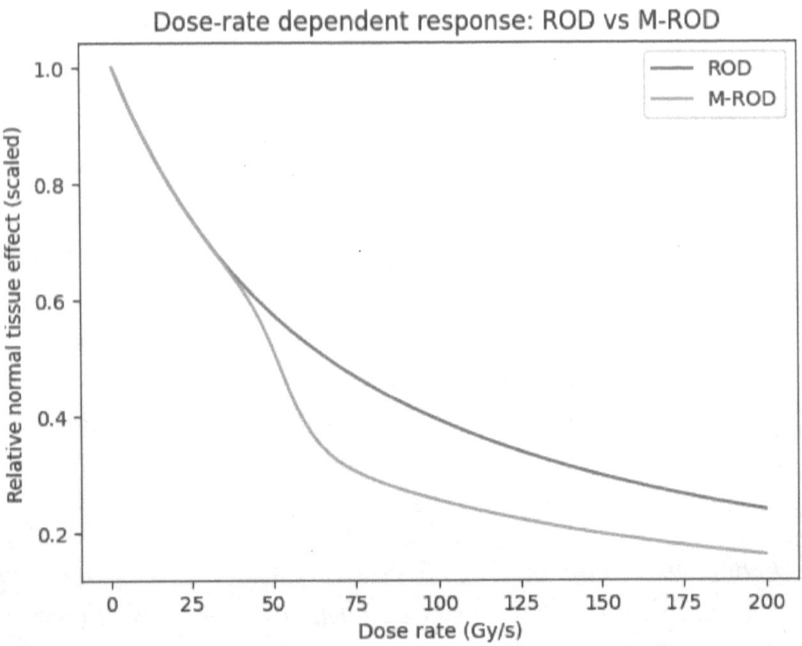

[Figure B2 — Relative normal tissue response vs dose rate. M-ROD shows threshold onset and saturation; ROD shows smooth continuous response. Source: Figure 2, Vaitheeswaran (2026b).]

Prediction 3: Pulse spacing determines biological outcome independently of total dose.

The History Rule (Rule 2) predicts path-dependence: the state trajectory depends on the timing of delivery, not only its total magnitude. M-ROD formalizes this through the decay term $-\gamma M$ — closely spaced pulses allow M to accumulate across successive pulses, amplifying protection; widely spaced pulses allow M to decay between pulses at rate γ, reducing cumulative activation. Figure B3 shows strong monotonic dependence of relative survival on inter-pulse interval in M-ROD, while ROD shows only weak dependence. This is the temporal structure signature. Crucially, total dose and average dose rate are held constant across all conditions — the only variable is pulse spacing.

Framework connection: Section A.3.2 — decay term -γM; Section A.10 — γ as the temporal decoherence parameter; History Rule (Rule 2).

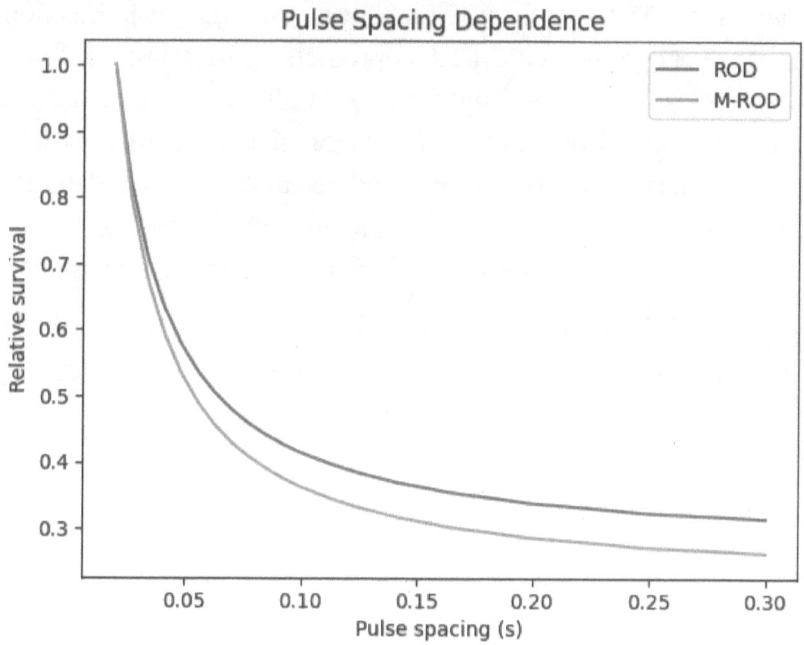

[Figure B3 — Relative survival vs pulse spacing. M-ROD shows strong inter-pulse interval sensitivity; ROD shows

weak dependence. Source: Figure 3, Vaitheeswaran (2026b).]

Prediction 4: Irradiation sequence changes biological outcome — the same total dose delivered in different temporal orders produces different results.

This is the purest expression of the History Rule: the state trajectory is path-dependent. Delivering high-dose-rate pulses first activates M(t) early, providing protection during subsequent low-dose-rate delivery. The reverse sequence activates M(t) late, providing less cumulative protection. Figure B4 shows that M-ROD predicts substantially different outcomes for Low→High versus High→Low sequences at identical total dose. ROD predicts identical outcomes for both — because it has no memory. This result directly validates the model's history-dependent architecture and provides a clean experimental discriminator between state-dependent and memoryless models.

Framework connection: Section A.3.2 — full M-ROD dynamics; History Rule (Rule 2); path-dependence as a framework prediction.

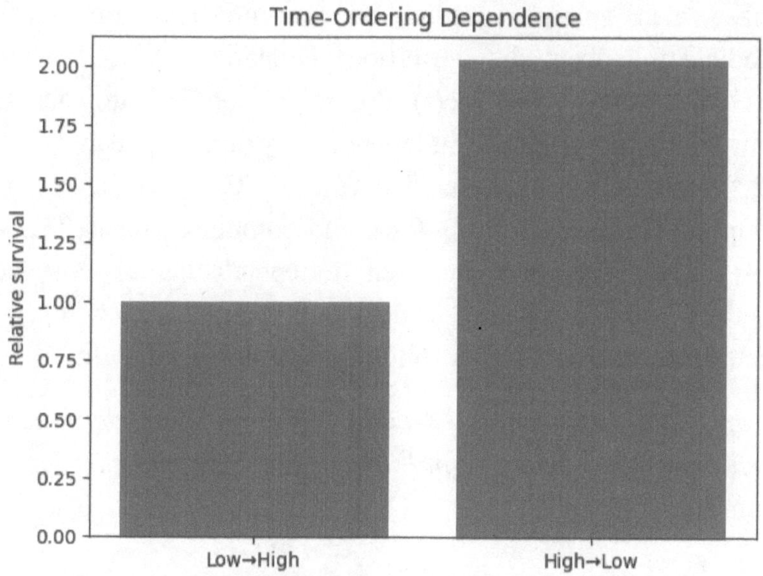

[Figure B4 — Time-ordering dependence. Low→High and High→Low sequences produce different outcomes in M-ROD, identical outcomes in ROD. Source: Figure 4, Vaitheeswaran (2026b).]

B.2 — TCI Framework: Spatial Coupling Detection (Vaitheeswaran, 2026a)

The TCI framework makes four predictions derivable from Section A.4. Each was tested in simulation under controlled coupling conditions.

Prediction 1: TCI is near zero under independence and rises specifically under spatial coupling.

If TCI correctly operationalizes the Interaction Rule, it must remain near zero when voxels evolve independently and rise only when spatial coupling is present. The framework predicts this from the definition: E_spatial ≈ E_ind when $x_i(t+1) \perp \{x_j(t)\}\_\{j \neq i\} \mid x_i(t)$. Figure B5 confirms this across four simulation regimes: independent dynamics (mean TCI ≈ 10^{-6}), temporal-only dynamics (mean TCI ≈ 10^{-6}), spatial coupling (mean TCI ≈ 0.3–0.4), and combined (mean TCI ≈ 0.3). The separation between independent and coupled regimes spans several orders of magnitude with no distributional overlap — strong discriminative capability.

Framework connection: Section A.4.3 — TCI definition; Section A.4.2 — mean signal invariance theorem; Interaction Rule (Rule 4).

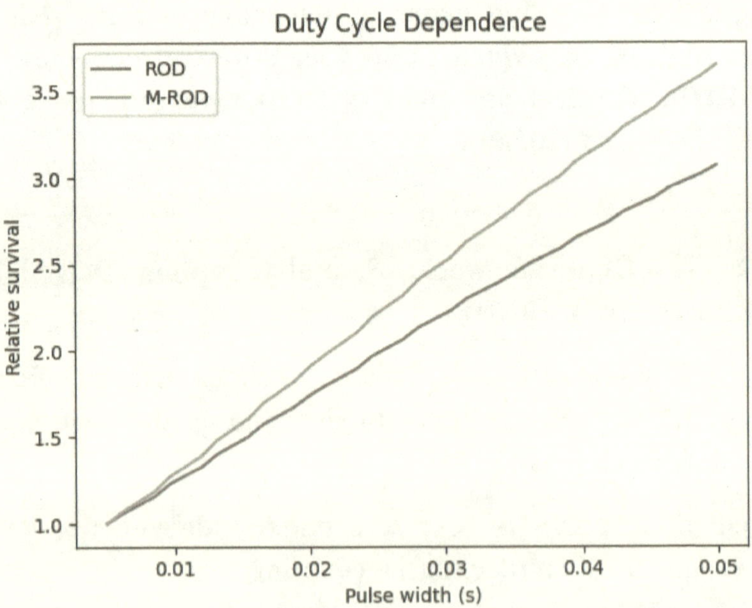

[Figure B5 — TCI across four simulation regimes. Independent and temporal-only conditions produce near-zero TCI; spatial and combined conditions produce substantially elevated TCI. Error bars show standard deviation across n=5 independent simulations. Source: Figure 1, Vaitheeswaran (2026a).]

Prediction 2: TCI collapses to near zero when structure is destroyed — confirming it detects genuine coupling rather than artifacts.

A metric that responds to noise or coincidental correlations would be clinically worthless. The framework requires that $TCI\_shuffled \approx 0$ when the spatiotemporal structure of the data is destroyed while preserving marginal distributions. Figure B6 shows that temporal shuffling and spatial randomization both collapse TCI from $\approx 0.4–0.5$ to $\approx 10^{-4}–10^{-3}$. The metric responds to genuine spatiotemporal structure, not to the marginal signal properties. This is the falsifiability condition the framework requires: a positive TCI is a positive finding, not a trivial artifact.

Framework connection: Section A.4.3 — falsifiability property; Observability Rule (Rule 6) — TCI as state observable.

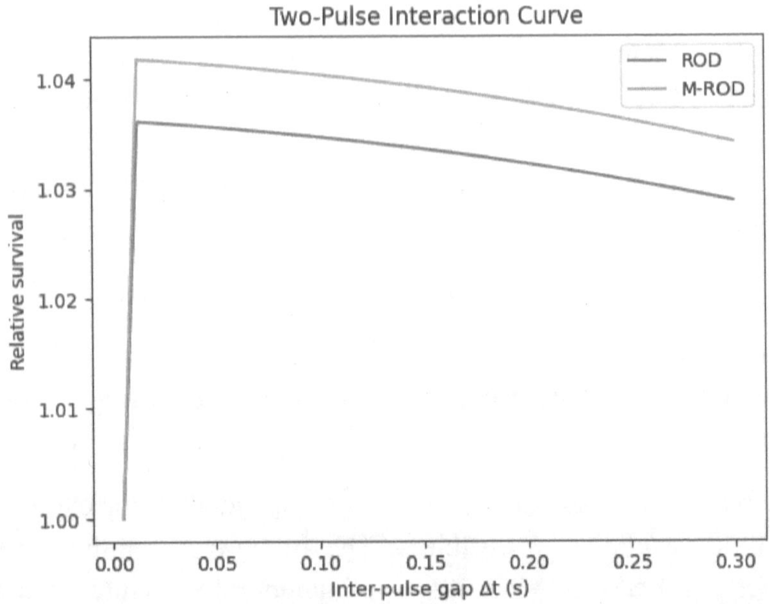

[Figure B6 — TCI under structure-destroying perturbations. Original structured dynamics yield high TCI; temporal and spatial shuffling collapse TCI to near zero. Source: Figure 2, Vaitheeswaran (2026a).]

Prediction 3: TCI increases monotonically with coupling strength.

The framework predicts from the eigenstructure analysis of Section A.4.4 that TCI is a monotonically increasing function of coupling strength D — stronger coupling produces larger eigenvalues in the coupling matrix, which contribute proportionally to TCI. Figure B7 confirms monotonic increase of TCI with D across the full range tested, with saturation at high coupling consistent with the regime in which voxel dynamics become highly correlated and additional spatial information becomes redundant. TCI is a continuous quantitative measure of interaction strength, not a binary indicator.

Framework connection: Section A.4.4 — TCI eigenstructure relationship; Interaction Rule (Rule 4) — coupling as causally active dimension of s_t.

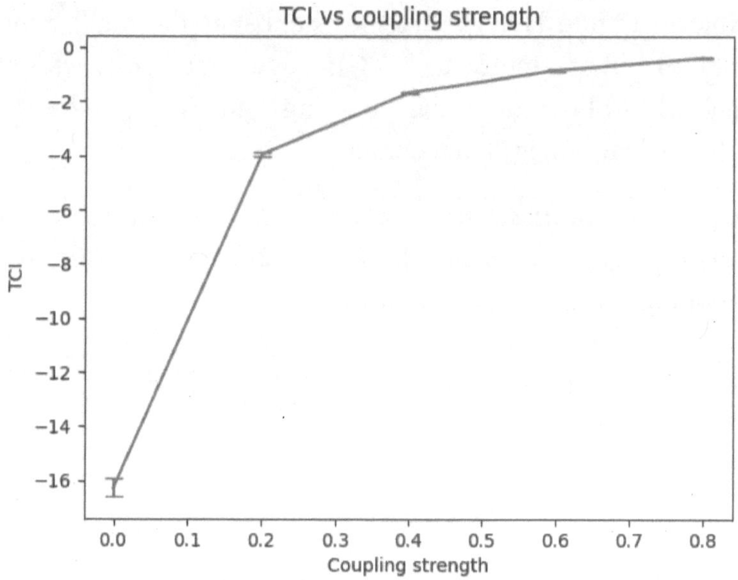

[Figure B7 — TCI vs spatial coupling strength D. Monotonic increase with saturation at high coupling. Error bars show standard deviation across n=5 simulations. Source: Figure 3, Vaitheeswaran (2026a).]

Prediction 4: Mean tumor signal is invariant to spatial coupling — the central identifiability result.

Section A.4.2 proves mathematically that the mean signal trajectory is independent of the coupling parameter λ by pairwise symmetry of the discrete Laplacian. This is not an approximation — it is exact for symmetric coupling matrices. Figure B8 demonstrates this computationally: mean signal trajectories for independent and strongly coupled systems (λ = 0.8) are visually indistinguishable across 100 time steps, despite dramatic differences in their internal spatial dynamics visible in Figure B9. This result establishes the fundamental limitation that motivates TCI: aggregate metrics are structurally blind to spatial coupling, and this blindness is mathematical rather than technical.

Framework connection: Section A.4.2 — mean signal invariance theorem (proved); Observability Rule (Rule 6) — partial observability as structural feature.

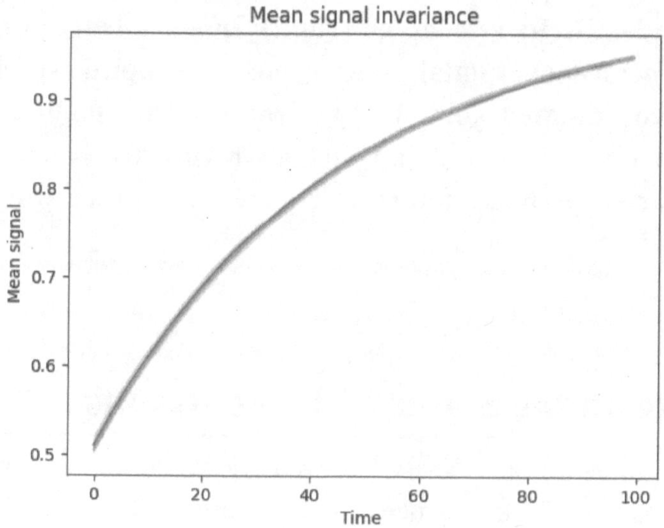

[Figure B8 — Mean tumor signal trajectories for independent (λ=0) and coupled (λ=0.8) systems. Trajectories are visually indistinguishable despite strong underlying spatial coupling. Source: Figure 4, Vaitheeswaran (2026a).]

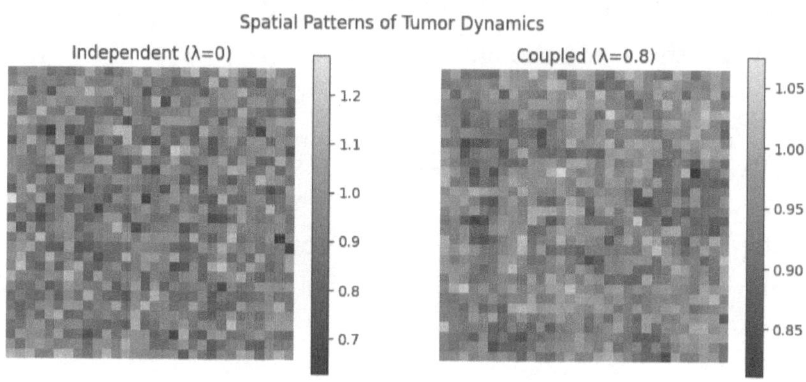

[Figure B9 — Spatial signal distribution at final time step: independent (left) vs coupled (right). Independent system shows persistent spatial heterogeneity; coupled system shows coordinated spatial organization. The qualitative difference invisible to mean metrics is directly visible in the spatial pattern. Source: Figure 5, Vaitheeswaran (2026a).]

A Note on the Status of These Results

Nine figures. Four M-ROD predictions and five TCI predictions, each confirmed in simulation. Together they establish that the model equations produce the behaviors the framework says they should produce under controlled conditions.

What they do not establish — and what no simulation study can establish — is that these behaviors occur in real tumors, in real patients, under real clinical conditions. The gap between a controlled simulation and a clinical trial is the gap between proof of principle and evidence. It is a gap that only prospective study can close.

These results are offered as the first step across that gap — not as the destination. The testable predictions in Appendix D specify what clinical data would be needed to take the next steps. Each figure in this appendix corresponds to at least one entry in Appendix D — a falsifiable prediction that real experiments can confirm or refute.

That is what a framework in its early life should produce. Not certainty. The right questions, asked precisely enough to get answered.

Appendix C
Connections to Parallel Theories

The informational state framework did not emerge in isolation. Three bodies of theory developed independently — in neuroscience, consciousness studies, and evolutionary oncology — converge on similar conclusions from different directions. This appendix maps those convergences precisely, states where they reinforce the informational state framework, and states honestly where they diverge or remain incompatible. The goal is not to claim that these theories validate each other — they do not, and conflating them would be intellectually dishonest — but to show that the informational state framework is part of a broader intellectual movement in biology toward organizational, systems-level, and information-theoretic descriptions of living systems.

C.1 — Integrated World Modeling Theory (IWMT)

Integrated World Modeling Theory, developed by Safron (2020, 2021), proposes that consciousness arises from the brain's capacity to construct hierarchical generative models of the world — models that integrate information across sensory modalities, temporal scales, and levels of abstraction into a unified predictive representation. The framework is grounded in the Free Energy Principle of Friston and colleagues, which the present book adopts in Chapters 13 and 15 as the normative framework for AIG-ART's inference architecture.

The convergence: IWMT treats the brain as a system that minimizes variational free energy by maintaining and updating a belief state over hidden causes of sensory data — exactly the architecture the AIG-ART framework applies to the tumor. In both cases, the hidden cause is an organizational state that is not directly observable, inference proceeds through a generative model that connects hidden states to observable consequences, and action is selected to minimize expected free energy. The mathematical structure is identical. The domain of application differs.

IWMT also emphasizes hierarchical organization — lower levels of the generative model are constrained by higher levels, and higher levels represent more abstract, integrated organizational properties. This maps directly onto the top-down causation argument of Chapters 9 and 10: the informational state s_t is a higher-level organizational representation that constrains lower-level cellular dynamics, exactly as higher levels of IWMT's generative model constrain lower-level sensory predictions.

The divergence: IWMT is a theory of conscious experience — its claims about phenomenal properties, subjective integration, and the relationship between information integration and awareness have no analog in the informational state framework. The tumor does not have a world model in any phenomenological sense. The AIG-ART framework borrows IWMT's mathematical architecture — hierarchical generative models, free energy minimization, belief updating

— without any of its claims about consciousness or subjective experience. The borrowing is technical, not conceptual.

C.2 — Integrated Information Theory (IIT)

Integrated Information Theory, developed by Tononi and colleagues (Tononi, 2004; Tononi et al., 2016), proposes that consciousness is identical to integrated information — a quantity Φ (phi) that measures how much information is generated by a system above and beyond the information generated by its parts independently. A system with high Φ has strong causal integration: its parts cannot be decomposed into independent subsystems without losing information. A system with low Φ is essentially decomposable — its parts operate independently.

The convergence: IIT's central concept — that causally integrated systems generate information that is irreducible to their parts — is the Interaction Rule (Rule 4) stated in information-theoretic language. A tumor with high TCI is a system in which voxel dynamics cannot be predicted independently without loss of predictive information — the spatial model improves over the independent model precisely because the system's parts are causally integrated. TCI is, in this sense, an operational cousin of Φ: both measure the extent to which a system's behavior exceeds what its parts independently predict.

The distinction between high-TCI and low-TCI tumors maps onto IIT's distinction between integrated and decomposable systems. A high-TCI tumor is one whose organizational state is irreducible — removing spatial information from the predictive model causes a measurable loss. A low-TCI tumor is approximately decomposable — its regions evolve near-independently.

IIT also emphasizes that integrated information is causally real — that Φ is not merely a description of the system but a measure of its causal power. This is the Constraint Rule (Rule 3) in information-theoretic form: the integrated organizational state exerts genuine causal influence on the system's dynamics, not reducible to the sum of independent component influences.

The divergence: IIT makes strong claims about consciousness — specifically that any system with $\Phi > 0$ has some degree of subjective experience. The informational state framework makes no such claim. More practically, Φ is computationally intractable for systems of any realistic size — its calculation requires evaluating all possible decompositions of the system, which scales super-exponentially with system size. TCI is computationally tractable by design: it requires only comparing two predictive models on observed data. TCI is therefore best understood as a clinically deployable approximation to the organizational integration that IIT formalizes — measuring the observable consequence of integration rather than integration itself.

C.3 — The Atavistic Theory of Cancer

The atavistic theory of cancer, developed primarily by Davies and Lineweaver (2011) and extended by Vincent (2012), proposes that cancer represents a partial reversion to evolutionarily ancient cellular programs — programs that predate the evolutionary invention of multicellular cooperation, in which individual cellular fitness and organismal fitness were one and the same. In the atavistic view, the suite of hallmarks of cancer — uncontrolled proliferation, invasion, evasion of cell death, metabolic reprogramming — are not random acquisitions but a coherent ancestral toolkit, latent in every cell's genome and suppressed in normal tissue by the organizational constraints of multicellular life.

The convergence: The atavistic theory provides the evolutionary context for the bioelectric biology of Chapter 10. The bioelectric organizational field — the tissue-wide pattern of membrane potentials that maintains spatial coherence and subordinates individual cell behavior to collective anatomical goals — is precisely the mechanism through which multicellular organisms suppress atavistic cellular programs. When the bioelectric field fails, as Chapter 10 established it does in cancer, the suppression is lifted and the ancient programs reassert themselves. Cancer, in both the atavistic theory and the informational state framework, is fundamentally a disease of organizational disruption — not of mutant molecules.

The atavistic theory also provides the deepest evolutionary grounding for the resistance-as-inference thread. Resistant cellular configurations are not novel evolutionary inventions — they are re-expressions of ancient programs whose fitness was high in the ancestral unicellular environment where individual cellular survival was the only evolutionary currency. These programs are already present in the genome of every cancer cell, suppressed by organizational constraints. Treatment pressure does not create resistance; it removes the organizational suppression that held it in check. This is competitive release — the evolutionary trap concept of Chapter 15 — stated in atavistic evolutionary terms.

The game-theoretic layer of AIG-ART is, from the atavistic perspective, a competition between the clinician's inference about the current organizational state and the ancient evolutionary programming of the tumor's cells attempting to re-express their atavistic fitness. The clinician's advantage is that they can reason prospectively about the tumor's evolutionary responses. The tumor's advantage is that its ancient programs have been optimized over billions of years of selection. The Stackelberg equilibrium is the policy that respects both.

The divergence: The atavistic theory makes specific claims about the genomic content of cancer cells — that the genes overexpressed in cancer are phylogenetically ancient, that they cluster in early-diverging branches of the eukaryotic tree of life, and that their expression levels correlate with cancer aggressiveness. These genomic predictions are not made by the informational state framework, which operates at the organizational level and makes no specific claims about which genes are expressed or how their evolutionary age relates to malignancy. The frameworks are complementary in their accounts of cancer's organizational character, but the atavistic theory's genomic claims require independent validation from evolutionary genomics, not from the informational state framework.

C.4 — Mukherjee's Organizational Picture of Cancer

Siddhartha Mukherjee is not a theorist in the sense that Friston, Tononi, or Davies and Lineweaver are theorists. He does not propose formal frameworks, derive equations, or make quantitative predictions. What he does — across three books spanning fifteen years of writing (Mukherjee, 2010, 2016, 2022) — is something equally important: he narrates the biological understanding of cancer with sufficient depth and honesty that the picture that emerges from his narrative converges, independently and without formal apparatus, on the same organizational description of cancer that the informational state framework formalizes.

This convergence is worth documenting precisely. It suggests that the organizational picture is not an artifact of the particular mathematical architecture chosen here but a genuine biological conclusion that multiple independent lines of inquiry are approaching from different directions.

The Emperor of All Maladies (2010) and the recurrence problem. Mukherjee's first book establishes the central clinical problem that motivates this framework: cancer returns in ways that the biology used to treat it cannot explain. His account of recurrence — of tumours that respond, appear controlled, and then reassert themselves in configurations that are resistant to the original treatment — is the clinical phenomenon that the informational state framework addresses formally. Mukherjee arrives at the conclusion that cancer is an evolutionary disease, that it adapts under selective pressure, and that treatment resistance is not random mutation but directed evolutionary response to clinical intervention. He stops at the evolutionary metaphor. The informational state framework continues: if cancer adapts evolutionarily, what is the organizational mechanism of that adaptation, and can it be formalized precisely enough to anticipate and intercept it? The Stackelberg game-theoretic layer of the AIG-ART framework is the formal answer to the question Mukherjee's narrative identifies but does not resolve.

The Gene (2016) and the limits of molecular reductionism. Mukherjee's second book argues, with great care and historical sweep, that the gene is not the sole determinant of biological outcome — that the same genetic sequence produces different phenotypes depending on context, history, and organizational state. His treatment of epigenetics is particularly relevant: he describes epigenetic marks as a layer of biological information that sits above the sequence and determines how the sequence is read, encoding developmental history in a form that persists without genomic change. This is the organizational layer that the informational state framework formalizes through the bioelectric state B_t and the clonal architecture E_t. Mukherjee does not give these dimensions a mathematical form — but his biological argument for their causal importance is precisely the argument that grounds the framework's claim that s_t is not reducible to molecular measurement.

The Song of the Cell (2022) and bioelectric organization. In his third book, Mukherjee arrives most directly at the biological substrate of the informational state framework. He devotes sustained attention to Michael Levin's work on bioelectric morphogenesis — the tissue-wide pattern of membrane potentials that governs how cells interpret their genetic instructions and maintain anatomical coherence across time. He describes the membrane potential as a kind of cellular memory, encoding organizational history in a form that persists without genomic change and that can be deliberately altered through physiological means. He writes about cancer as a disease in which this organizational memory is disrupted — cells that have lost access to the global bioelectric information that maintains their subordination to the purposes of the whole. This is, stated in narrative rather than mathematical language, exactly the bioelectric state B_t component of the informational state, and exactly the top-down causation argument of Chapters 9 and 10 of this book. Mukherjee intuited the clinical importance of this layer. The Ghost in the Cancer formalizes it and asks what it implies for how radiation interacts with organized versus disorganized tissue.

The nature of the convergence. Mukherjee's three books, read in sequence, trace an intellectual journey from molecular reductionism toward organizational complexity — from the gene as the unit of biological information toward the cell, the tissue, and the bioelectric field as equally important levels of organization. By the end of *The Song of the Cell*, the organizational picture of cancer that the informational state framework formalizes is clearly visible in Mukherjee's narrative — not as a formal theory but as a biological conclusion that his careful engagement with the experimental literature has made unavoidable.

The informational state framework is, in a precise sense, the clinical theory that Mukherjee's biological narrative has been building toward without quite arriving at. It takes the organizational picture of cancer that three books of careful synthesis have established and asks the question that narrative alone cannot answer: given that this picture is correct, what should a radiotherapy system do differently, and how should it do it?

C.5 — What the Convergences Mean

Four independent intellectual traditions have arrived, through entirely different methods, at the same organizational picture of cancer. A consciousness theorist working from the mathematics of information integration. A physicist working from the thermodynamics of self-organizing systems. An evolutionary biologist working from the deep history of multicellular life. A physician-writer working from fifteen years of careful engagement with the experimental literature of cancer biology. None of them set out to converge. And yet each arrives, in their own language, at the same conclusion: that cancer is fundamentally a failure of organizational coherence rather than a failure of molecular fidelity, and that understanding and treating it requires engaging with organizational structure directly rather than reducing it to molecular components.

The convergence is not coincidental. It reflects something genuine about the biology.

But every one of these arguments was made from inference. Theoretical necessity. Developmental biology in model organisms. Accumulated experimental observation pointing consistently in one direction. Davies and Lineweaver (2011) argued the organizational picture from evolutionary necessity.

Levin (2021) argued it from bioelectric developmental biology. Mukherjee (2022) argued it from three decades of clinical-biological synthesis. Tononi et al. (2016) and Safron (2020, 2021) argued the causal reality of integrated organizational states from the mathematics of information and consciousness. Each argument is compelling. None had direct experimental demonstration that a non-neural biological network learns associations, that this learning is measurable as a structural reorganization rather than merely a behavioral change, and that the learned state can be selectively erased without disrupting the network's architecture or its capacity to learn again.

That demonstration now exists. Pigozzi et al. (2025) showed that gene regulatory networks undergo associative conditioning in the precise Pavlovian sense — and that the conditioning increases causal emergence, making the network's behavior more governed by its collective state and less by the independent dynamics of its parts. Learning, in biological networks, reorganizes rather than merely records. Doan et al. (2026) showed the same capacity for associative memory in *Stentor coeruleus*, a single-celled organism with no nervous system, establishing that this is a general property of biological dynamical systems rather than a specialization of complex multicellular networks. The selective erasure result of Pigozzi et al. (2025) demonstrated further that memory encoded as organizational state can be deliberately disrupted and redirected through targeted intervention — without structural damage to the network itself.

These results were not available to any of the predecessor works discussed in this appendix. They transform the organizational picture of cancer from a conclusion argued by inference into a conclusion supported by direct experimental demonstration. And they carry a specific implication that none of the predecessor frameworks could have drawn: if biological networks learn in this precise, experimentally demonstrated sense, then a tumor under repeated radiation exposure is not merely adapting stochastically under selective pressure. It is integrating the information content of the treatment being applied and reorganizing its internal configuration in ways that reflect what it has learned. Resistance is not only an evolutionary phenomenon. It is a learning phenomenon. And learning, as Pigozzi et al. (2025) demonstrated, leaves a specific organizational signature — rising causal emergence, increasing integration of the network's parts — that is in principle detectable before it is detectable as clinical treatment failure.

Each tradition contributes something the others do not. IIT contributes the proof that organizational integration is causally irreducible. IWMT contributes the mathematical architecture for acting under partial observability. The Atavistic Theory contributes the evolutionary grounding for resistance as organizational reversion. Mukherjee contributes the clinical-biological validation that the organizational picture is not theoretical abstraction but a conclusion forced by the experimental literature of cancer itself. And the experimental record of Pigozzi et al. (2025) and Doan et al. (2026) contributes what none of the others could: direct demonstration that biological networks learn, that learning reorganizes organizational structure in a measurable way, and that the learned state can in principle be disrupted.

What none of these traditions contributes, individually or together, is clinical specificity. IIT does not tell you what to do with a strongly coupled tumour. IWMT does not specify a dose prescription. The Atavistic Theory does not design a treatment policy. Mukherjee does not derive a generalized radiobiological model. The convergence establishes that the organizational picture is correct and important. The experimental record establishes that biological networks learn and that their learning is organizationally visible. This book is the first to ask what a radiotherapy machine should do about both facts simultaneously — and to build the answer with enough mathematical precision and clinical specificity to be tested.

The epistemological diversity of the five traditions is not a weakness of the convergence but its greatest strength. A conclusion forced by deductive mathematics, confirmed by evolutionary biology, validated by experimental cancer biology, demonstrated directly in biological network learning experiments, and made clinically operational by a formal treatment framework is not an artifact of any particular method. It is a feature of the world.

Whether the informational state framework correctly characterizes that feature belongs to the experiments of Appendix D. The traditions have established that the organizational picture is worth formalizing. The experimental record has established that biological networks learn in ways that leave organizational signatures. Whether this formalization correctly captures both — and whether the clinical tools proposed here detect what they claim to detect — is an empirical question. It has an empirical answer.

The conversation is not ending here. It is just becoming precise enough to be tested.

Appendix D
Testable Predictions Register

A framework earns its place in science not through elegance but through exposure. This appendix states the framework's predictions with enough precision that they can be tested, and enough honesty that they can be falsified.

One criterion governs every entry: the prediction must be genuinely new — something no competing framework generates — and the experiment must be achievable with equipment and infrastructure that exists today. Predictions that follow from mathematical necessity alone, or that could be derived from existing frameworks without invoking the informational state, are not listed here. What is listed are the studies that could begin now, at institutions already equipped with MR-linac systems, FLASH-capable accelerators, liquid biopsy programmes, and tumour organoid facilities. The gap between this register and the vision of Chapter 17 is not a gap of imagination. It is a gap of validation — and closing it is the work of the next decade.

The predictions are organised in two tiers. Tier 2 predictions are testable in controlled laboratory or early clinical studies with currently available equipment, each specific to a model component and falsifiable without large clinical trials. Tier 3 predictions require prospective clinical studies; falsifying any of them forces fundamental revision of the framework's core claims. Each prediction states what should be observed if the framework is correct, what should be observed if it is wrong, and what study would decide between them.

A note on confidence: not all predictions carry equal weight. Three of the nine — T2.1, T2.5, and T3.1 — are the framework's highest-stakes claims. No competing framework generates them. If all three are positive, the informational state framework has earned its place. If any is decisively negative, the framework requires fundamental revision. The remaining four predictions test specific components — the bioelectric coherence hierarchy, the oxygen-memory coupling mechanism, the bioelectric field modulation, and the causal priority of clonal over organisational dynamics. Each is genuinely new; each tests a specific architectural element rather than the framework as a whole.

Tier 2 — Model-Specific Predictions

These are testable in controlled laboratory or early clinical studies with currently available equipment. Each is specific to a model component and falsifiable without large clinical trials.

T2.1 — Pulse-spacing dependence at fixed total dose and average dose rate

This is the single most important near-term experimental test of the M-ROD model.

Statement: Delivering identical total dose at identical average dose rate through pulsed FLASH irradiation, while systematically varying the inter-pulse interval, will produce significantly different biological outcomes. Closely spaced pulses — within $1/\gamma$ of each other — produce greater normal tissue protection. Widely spaced pulses — separated by multiples of $1/\gamma$ — produce progressively less protection as M(t) decays between pulses. The protective effect should scale approximately as $\exp(-\gamma\Delta t)$ relative to the maximum protection achieved at $\Delta t \to 0$.

What falsifies it: No significant difference in clonogenic survival or tissue damage across pulse spacings when total dose and average dose rate are matched. Classical ROD predicts this null result. If the null result is obtained in a properly controlled experiment, the M-ROD memory mechanism does not operate.

Why this is new: The existence of pulse-spacing effects in FLASH has been observed in preliminary work. What no experiment has done is systematically vary pulse spacing at rigorously matched total dose and average dose rate, measure the differential sparing factor across a range of intervals, and test the fit of the $\exp(-\gamma\Delta t)$ functional form against a measurable M-ROD parameter. The quantitative prediction of a specific functional form tied to a specific parameter is what distinguishes this from prior work and from what classical ROD predicts.

Proposed experiment: In vitro clonogenic survival assay using normal tissue cell lines — lung fibroblasts, intestinal organoids — irradiated with FLASH electron beams at matched total dose (10 Gy) and average dose rate (50 Gy/s), with inter-pulse intervals of 10, 50, 100, 200, and 300 ms. Simultaneously irradiate matched tumour cell lines. Measure differential sparing factor — ratio of normal tissue survival to tumour survival — at each pulse spacing. M-ROD predicts a monotonically falling sparing factor as pulse spacing increases, with the inflection point at approximately $1/\gamma$ seconds. ROD predicts no significant trend.

Infrastructure required: FLASH-capable electron accelerator (operational at multiple centres); standard clonogenic assay. Achievable within six months at any FLASH-equipped radiobiology laboratory.

T2.2 — Time-ordering sensitivity is tissue-specific and follows the bioelectric coherence hierarchy

Statement: M-ROD predicts that time-ordering sensitivity — the degree to which high-to-low versus low-to-high dose rate sequences produce different outcomes — is greatest in tissues with the highest bioelectric organisational coherence. The framework predicts a specific tissue hierarchy: cardiac muscle (highest connexin-43 density) > intestinal epithelium > lung parenchyma > tumour tissue (lowest coherence, least time-ordering sensitivity).

What falsifies it: Time-ordering sensitivity is tissue-independent — cardiac muscle and tumour tissue show equivalent sensitivity to irradiation sequence at matched dose and dose rate. Or the hierarchy is inverted.

Why this is new: Time-ordering sensitivity has been observed but never systematically compared across tissue types in a way that tests a specific hierarchy derived from bioelectric coherence. The prediction of a specific tissue ranking — derived from connexin-43 density as a proxy for organisational coherence — is entirely new. A flat hierarchy falsifies the bioelectric coherence coupling. An inverted hierarchy falsifies M-ROD entirely. Both failure modes are informative in specific directions.

Proposed experiment: Ex vivo tissue irradiation using cardiac, lung, intestinal, and tumour tissue samples. Deliver matched total dose (8 Gy) at matched average dose rate (60 Gy/s) in two sequences: high-to-low (initial 100 Gy/s followed by 20 Gy/s completion) and low-to-high (reversed). Measure DNA double-strand break repair kinetics (γH2AX foci at 30 min and 4 h) as a proxy for biological effectiveness. M-ROD predicts the differential between sequences will rank in the bioelectric coherence hierarchy.

Infrastructure required: FLASH-capable electron accelerator; standard immunofluorescence for γH2AX. Achievable at any FLASH-equipped centre with access to ex vivo tissue samples.

T2.3 — Real-time oxygen dynamics during FLASH delivery follow M-ROD predictions and differ between tumour and normal tissue

---

Statement: The M-ROD model makes specific predictions about the temporal profile of oxygen concentration O(t) during and immediately after FLASH delivery — specifically, that O(t) drops sharply during the pulse cluster, recovers at a rate governed by the tissue's vascular reperfusion capacity, and that the shape of the O(t) recovery curve — specifically its initial slope and time-to-half-recovery — differs systematically between tumour tissue and organised normal tissue in a manner consistent with their respective bioelectric coherence states. This differential will correlate with the degree of FLASH-mediated normal tissue sparing observed in the same tissue samples.

What falsifies it: The O(t) recovery profile is indistinguishable between tumour and normal tissue at matched oxygenation levels. Or the photoacoustic signal does not correlate with the biological sparing effect — meaning oxygen dynamics are decoupled from tissue protection. Either result forces revision of the oxygen-memory coupling mechanism at the heart of M-ROD.

Why this is new: Photoacoustic imaging of oxygen dynamics during FLASH has been proposed as a measurement approach. What is new is the specific claim about the shape of O(t) recovery — not just its magnitude — and the cross-validation against T2.1: M-ROD parameters fitted from the pulse-spacing experiment (T2.1) should independently predict the O(t) recovery profile measured here without additional fitting. This cross-experiment parameter consistency is the uniquely framework-derived test.

Proposed experiment: Ex vivo tissue preparation using matched tumour and normal tissue samples — lung, intestinal, and tumour xenograft. Mount samples in a photoacoustic imaging chamber with simultaneous FLASH electron beam delivery capability. Deliver 10 Gy at 60 Gy/s and acquire photoacoustic oxygen maps at 10 ms intervals for

2 seconds before, during, and 30 seconds after delivery. Extract O(t) curves for each tissue type. Fit M-ROD oxygen dynamics equations to the measured curves and compare fitted parameters — depletion rate, recovery half-time — against model predictions derived independently from the T2.1 pulse-spacing experiment. Simultaneously measure clonogenic survival to correlate O(t) differential with biological sparing differential.

Infrastructure required: FLASH-capable electron accelerator; photoacoustic imaging system with millisecond temporal resolution; ex vivo tissue preparation facility. This experiment requires co-location of FLASH delivery and photoacoustic imaging — a non-trivial engineering constraint but achievable at centres with FLASH-equipped radiobiology laboratories. Estimated timeline: twelve months from equipment co-location to first results.

T2.4 — Bioelectric field application modifies TCI in a frequency-dependent and reversible manner

Statement: External alternating electric fields modulate gap junctional conductance and thereby TCI. Intermediate-frequency fields (100–300 kHz, the TTFields range) will reduce TCI in tumour organoid models by disrupting gap junctional connectivity. Low-frequency fields (1–10 Hz) will have minimal effect. The effect should be reversible — TCI should recover when the field is removed.

What falsifies it: Electric field application at any frequency produces no significant change in TCI measured from tumour organoid imaging. Or the effect is not reversible, suggesting permanent structural disruption rather than dynamic modulation.

What this prediction tests: This is a component validation — it tests the bioelectric field modulation mechanism (the B_t control dimension), not the framework as a whole. TTFields are known to affect gap junctional connectivity, so the existence of an effect is not new. What is new is framing the result as a TCI modification and predicting the frequency-dependent pattern. A positive result validates the most speculative control dimension of AIG-ART. A null result indicates that the B_t dimension as conceived does not operate and must be revised or removed. The experiment required to validate or refute the clinical bioelectric modulation claim is this one — referenced throughout the book as Appendix D prediction T2.4.

Proposed experiment: 3D tumour organoid models imaged with serial optical coherence tomography or confocal microscopy to generate the voxel-level temporal dynamics required for TCI computation. Apply TTFields at 100, 200, and 300 kHz, and low-frequency fields at 1, 5, and 10 Hz, for two hours each. Compute TCI before, during, and 24 hours after field application. Simultaneously measure connexin-43 expression and membrane potential using voltage-sensitive dye imaging.

Infrastructure required: TTFields device (Optune, FDA-approved and clinically available); tumour organoid culture facility; serial high-resolution optical imaging for TCI computation. The imaging modality is the technical constraint — standard clinical imaging lacks the spatial resolution and temporal frequency required for TCI in organoids. This experiment requires a specialist cell imaging facility.

T2.5 — A sub-therapeutic probing pulse generates state-discriminating observations that predict subsequent therapeutic response

This prediction is the most distinctively new in the register. No competing framework generates it.

Statement: A sub-therapeutic radiation pulse (0.1–0.3 Gy) delivered at the start of a treatment fraction — before the therapeutic dose — generates a multi-modal biological response that differs systematically between tumours in different organisational states. Specifically, the spatial pattern of the ADC response to the probing pulse at fraction one will predict which tumour subregions respond to subsequent SFRT delivery and which do not, independent of the baseline ADC value.

What falsifies it: The probing pulse response pattern adds no predictive information about subsequent treatment response beyond what baseline ADC and TCI alone provide. The spatial response to a 0.1 Gy pulse is indistinguishable from noise at clinically relevant imaging resolutions.

Why this is new: No existing radiobiological framework predicts that a sub-therapeutic pulse carries state-discriminating information. The classical framework treats dose below the therapeutic threshold as biologically inert — producing no relevant response and carrying no information about the tumour's internal state. The informational state framework predicts the opposite: the tumour's response to even a minimal perturbation reflects its current organisational configuration, and that reflection is spatially structured in a way that predicts how it will respond to therapeutic perturbations. A positive result — spatial probing pulse response predicts SFRT response independently of baseline ADC — would be inexplicable without the informational state concept. There is no available alternative explanation.

Proposed experiment: In patients treated on MR-linac for locally advanced rectal or cervical cancer, deliver a 0.1 Gy probing pulse at the start of fraction one, followed by standard therapeutic delivery. Acquire DWI immediately before and 30 minutes after the probing pulse. Compute the spatial pattern of the ADC response. At the end of the treatment course, assess whether the spatial probing pulse response predicts the spatial pattern of pathological response. Compare predictive power against baseline ADC alone and TCI alone. The incremental dose from the probing pulse (0.1 Gy) is less than 0.5% of a standard 60 Gy course — within the dose uncertainty that adaptive radiotherapy already accepts routinely.

Infrastructure required: MR-linac with DWI capability; no additional hardware. The probing pulse is within the linac's existing delivery capability.

Tier 3 — Framework-Level Predictions

These require prospective clinical studies. Falsifying any of them forces fundamental revision of the framework's core claims. All three are feasible with currently existing clinical infrastructure.

T3.1 — TCI trajectory inflection point precedes clinical resistance detection by at least two fractions

This is the framework's primary clinical validation prediction.

Statement: In patients who develop local recurrence or pathological non-response after radiotherapy, TCI will show a reversal — rising after an initial decline — at least two treatment fractions before conventional imaging metrics (mean ADC, SUV, tumour volume) show any sign of inadequate response.

The two-fraction minimum lead time is derived from the model: organisational reorganisation must precede detectable metabolic or volumetric change, because organisational state changes drive the metabolic and proliferative changes that eventually produce imaging-detectable consequences. The lead time is not a free parameter — it is a structural consequence of the causal hierarchy in the framework.

What falsifies it: TCI reversal does not occur more frequently in non-responders than responders. Or TCI reversal occurs simultaneously with or after conventional metric changes — indicating that TCI is tracking the same events as conventional imaging rather than a causally upstream organisational state.

Why this is new: TCI itself is new. The prediction of a specific lead time — minimum two fractions — derived from the causal structure of the model is new. No existing framework predicts that an organisational metric will precede metabolic response; existing adaptive radiotherapy frameworks treat imaging metrics as concurrent rather than causally upstream. A positive result means the framework's central causal claim — that organisational state changes drive, rather than accompany, treatment failure — is supported with clinically measurable precision.

Proposed study: Prospective observational cohort on MR-linac, minimum 80 patients, disease sites with high local recurrence rates — rectal cancer, cervical cancer, head-and-neck. Daily ADC imaging with TCI computation at every fraction. Primary endpoint: fraction at which TCI reversal occurs versus fraction at which mean ADC plateaus, in patients who achieve pathological complete response versus those who do not. Powered to detect a two-fraction lead time with 80% power.

Infrastructure required: MR-linac with daily DWI; TCI computation software; pathological response assessment at surgery. No new hardware. Feasible at any MR-linac centre treating rectal or cervical cancer.

T3.2 — EIT impedance signatures during radiotherapy precede ADC changes and provide independent predictive information

Statement: Serial EIT measurements acquired during a course of MR-linac radiotherapy will: (i) provide independent predictive information about local control and recurrence beyond what ADC trajectory alone provides; (ii) show characteristic impedance shifts at least one fraction before the corresponding ADC change becomes significant; and (iii) show differential impedance trajectories between tumour subregions that subsequently show coordinated versus independent ADC dynamics — providing an independent, non-MRI window into the spatial organisational structure that TCI captures from ADC data.

What falsifies it: Serial EIT adds no independent predictive information about local control beyond what ADC trajectory provides in a multivariate model. Or EIT impedance changes occur simultaneously with or after ADC changes — indicating that EIT is tracking the same biological events as MRI rather than a causally upstream organisational state.

What this prediction tests: The general claim that EIT adds value to radiotherapy monitoring is not uniquely this framework's prediction — other frameworks invoking bioelectric state would generate it. What is uniquely framework-derived is the lead-time prediction: that EIT precedes ADC because EIT tracks the bioelectric organisational state, which is causally upstream of the metabolic changes ADC measures. The lead-time sub-prediction is the discriminating test.

Proposed study: Prospective observational cohort of 60 patients treated on MR-linac for locally advanced rectal or cervical cancer. EIT electrodes applied at each fraction using a sixteen-electrode belt system positioned around the pelvis. Acquire EIT at three time points per fraction: immediately before, during, and thirty minutes after delivery. Extract spatial impedance maps and compute: (i) mean impedance trajectory per tumour subregion; (ii) inter-subregion impedance correlation; (iii) timing of first significant impedance shift relative to first significant ADC shift. Primary endpoint: partial R^2 of EIT trajectory in a multivariate model predicting pathological complete response, after controlling for ADC trajectory, tumour volume, and clinical staging. Secondary endpoint: lead time of EIT change over ADC change in non-responders.

Infrastructure required: MR-linac with daily DWI (as in T3.1); MR-compatible EIT system — commercially available from Swisstom and Dräger, with carbon-fibre electrodes to avoid susceptibility artefacts. No new clinical protocols beyond T3.1; EIT adds a non-ionising measurement with no incremental patient risk.

T3.3 — ctDNA clonal monitoring detects emerging resistance at least two fractions before TCI reversal

Statement: Because clonal selection drives organisational reorganisation — not the reverse — the ctDNA signal should precede the TCI reversal signal. In patients who subsequently show TCI reversal (as detected by T3.1), the ctDNA clonal fraction of treatment-resistant subpopulations will have been rising for at least two fractions before TCI reversal becomes detectable.

What falsifies it: TCI reversal and ctDNA clonal shift occur simultaneously. Or TCI reversal precedes the ctDNA signal — which would invert the causal direction the framework proposes and indicate that organisational reorganisation is not driven by clonal selection.

Why this is new: The prediction of a specific two-fraction lead time in a specific causal direction — ctDNA before TCI, because clonal dynamics drive organisational state, not the reverse — is new. It makes a testable causal claim about the relationship between two different measurement modalities, both novel in this context, and specifies which should move first. A result showing simultaneous movement weakens the causal claim. A result showing TCI moving first would force revision of the framework's causal architecture.

Proposed study: Nested within the T3.1 study, adding per-fraction liquid biopsy to the existing protocol. Incremental cost is the liquid biopsy processing; no additional imaging or delivery infrastructure is required. Primary analysis compares the timing of ctDNA clonal shift against TCI reversal in the same patients.

Infrastructure required: MR-linac (as in T3.1); liquid biopsy and clonal fraction analysis. Feasible as a nested study at centres with liquid biopsy capability.

T3.4 — A ctDNA-guided adaptive policy outperforms standard dose escalation specifically in patients with detectable resistant clone at baseline

Statement: In oligometastatic prostate cancer with identifiable sensitive and resistant clonal populations at baseline ctDNA, a treatment policy that moderates dose to regions harbouring the sensitive clone — deliberately maintaining its population as a competitive suppressor of the resistant clone — will produce longer progression-free survival than a standard maximum-dose policy. In patients with homogeneous sensitive tumours (no detectable resistant clone at baseline), the two policies will produce equivalent outcomes.

The critical prediction is not that lower total dose is generally better — it is the interaction term: benefit from adaptive policy only in the heterogeneous stratum. This interaction is the uniquely framework-derived element. Without the informational state framework's account of competitive suppression through organisational coupling, you would not predict that this specific patient subgroup benefits while the homogeneous subgroup does not.

What falsifies it: The ctDNA-guided adaptive policy produces equivalent or inferior progression-free survival across all patients. Or the policy × baseline clonal heterogeneity interaction term is non-significant — meaning the framework's prediction of subgroup-specific benefit is wrong. A null result on the interaction term would indicate that the competitive suppression mechanism, as modelled here, does not operate in this clinical context.

Proposed study: Randomised phase II trial in oligometastatic prostate cancer — three or fewer metastatic sites — concurrent with androgen deprivation therapy. Stratify by baseline ctDNA clonal heterogeneity (homogeneous sensitive versus detectable resistant clone present). Randomise within each stratum to ctDNA-guided adaptive radiotherapy versus standard SBRT at maximum tolerated dose. Primary endpoint: 18-month progression-free survival. Key secondary endpoint: policy × baseline clonal heterogeneity interaction term. The framework predicts benefit from the adaptive policy only in the heterogeneous stratum. A significant interaction in the predicted direction, with equivalent outcomes in the homogeneous stratum, would validate the competitive suppression mechanism.

Infrastructure required: SBRT-capable linac; per-fraction liquid biopsy with rapid clonal fraction turnaround (24 hours). Several academic cancer centres currently have this capability.

The Priority Order

If resources permitted only one experiment from this register, it should be **T2.1** — the pulse-spacing dependence experiment. Achievable in six months with existing FLASH equipment, requiring no patients, generating a clean binary result: M-ROD is either right or wrong about the specific functional form of its central prediction.

If resources permitted a second experiment, it should be **T2.5** — the probing pulse state discrimination experiment. It requires only an MR-linac with standard DWI, tests the most distinctively new prediction in the register, and produces a result no alternative framework can explain if positive.

The natural sequence that follows:

— T2.1 and T2.5 positive → proceed to T2.2 (tissue hierarchy) and T2.3 (photoacoustic O(t))

— T3.1 designed and recruiting → T3.2 added as parallel EIT cohort; T3.3 nested within T3.1 as liquid biopsy add-on

— T3.1 positive and T3.3 positive → proceed to T3.4 (adaptive trial) if liquid biopsy infrastructure and clonal fraction turnaround are available

— T2.4 (bioelectric field modulation) proceeds in parallel with the clinical programme — it requires specialist cell imaging infrastructure but not clinical trial approval

A Final Note

This register will age. Some predictions will be confirmed before this book reaches its second printing. Others will be falsified and will require the framework to be revised. Some experiments proposed here will be superseded by better designs.

The register is not a monument. It is a working document, and its most important property is not the elegance of its predictions but the honesty with which it invites their refutation. The framework does not need to be right about everything. It needs to be right about enough — and wrong in ways that teach us something — to have earned its place in the scientific conversation about cancer and its control.

The three predictions that matter most — T2.1, T2.5, and T3.1 — are the ones where the informational state framework stands alone. No existing radiobiological framework predicts pulse-spacing dependence with a specific functional form. No existing framework predicts that a sub-therapeutic pulse carries state-discriminating spatial information. No existing framework predicts that an organisational coupling metric precedes clinical resistance by a specific lead time derived from a causal model. These three predictions are where the framework commits. That conversation is just beginning.

List of Acronyms

Acronym	Full Form
ABR	Auditory Brainstem Response
ADC	Apparent Diffusion Coefficient
AIG-ART	Active Inference-Guided Adaptive Radiotherapy
CBCT	Cone Beam Computed Tomography
CELI	Cherenkov-Excited Luminescence Imaging
CPU/GPU	Central/Graphics Processing Unit
CT	Computed Tomography
ctDNA	Circulating Tumour DNA
D	Dose (Gray)
DNA	Deoxyribonucleic Acid
DSB	Double-Strand Break
DWI	Diffusion-Weighted Imaging
EIT	Electrical Impedance Tomography
FDG	Fluorodeoxyglucose
FEP	Free Energy Principle
fNIRS	Functional Near-Infrared Spectroscopy
GRN	Gene Regulatory Network

Gy	Gray (unit of absorbed radiation dose)
Gy/s	Gray per second (dose rate)
Hill	Hill function (sigmoidal activation)
IGRT	Image-Guided Radiotherapy
IMPT	Intensity-Modulated Proton Therapy
IMRT	Intensity-Modulated Radiotherapy
IIT	Integrated Information Theory
IWMT	Integrated World Modeling Theory
KL	Kullback-Leibler (divergence)
LAD	Left Anterior Descending (coronary artery)
LET	Linear Energy Transfer
LKB	Lyman-Kutcher-Burman (NTCP model)
LQ	Linear-Quadratic (model)
M-ROD	Memory-modulated Radiolytic Oxygen Depletion
MACE	Major Adverse Cardiac Event
MR	Magnetic Resonance
MR-linac	Magnetic Resonance Linear Accelerator
MRI	Magnetic Resonance Imaging
NIR	Near-Infrared

NTCP	Normal Tissue Complication Probability
OAR	Organ At Risk
PACT	Photoacoustic Computed Tomography
PET	Positron Emission Tomography
POMDP	Partially Observable Markov Decision Process
RBE	Relative Biological Effectiveness
ROD	Radiolytic Oxygen Depletion
SBRT	Stereotactic Body Radiotherapy
SFRT	Spatially Fractionated Radiotherapy
SF	Surviving Fraction
SUV	Standardised Uptake Value
TCP	Tumour Control Probability
TCI	Tumour Coupling Index
TTFields	Tumour Treating Fields

References

Alon, U. (2007). An Introduction to Systems Biology: Design Principles of Biological Circuits. Chapman & Hall/CRC.

Antonuk, L. E. (2002). Electronic portal imaging devices: a review & historical perspective of contemporary technologies & research. Physics in Medicine & Biology, 47(6), R31–R65.

Antonuk, L. E., Boudry, J., Huang, W., McShan, D. L., Morton, E. J., Yorkston, J., Longo, M. J., & Street, R. A. (1992). Demonstration of megavoltage & diagnostic x-ray imaging with hydrogenated amorphous silicon arrays. Medical Physics, 19(6), 1455–1466.

Astrahan, M. A. (2008). Some implications of linear-quadratic-linear radiation dose-response with regard to hypofractionation. Medical Physics, 35(9), 4161–4172.

Barabási, A. L., & Oltvai, Z. N. (2004). Network biology: understanding the cell's functional organization. Nature Reviews Genetics, 5(2), 101–113.

Beal, M. J. (2003). Variational algorithms for approximate Bayesian inference. PhD Thesis, University College London.

Beane, W. S., et al. (2011). A chemical genetics approach reveals H,K-ATPase-mediated membrane voltage is required for planarian head regeneration. Chemical Biology, 18(1), 77–89.

Bellman, R., & Åström, K. J. (1970). On structural identifiability. Mathematical Biosciences, 7(3–4), 329–339.

Bernier, J., Hall, E. J., & Giaccia, A. (2004). Radiation oncology: a century of achievements. Nature Reviews Cancer, 4(9), 737–747.

Bertalanffy, L. von (1968). General System Theory: Foundations, Development, Applications. George Braziller.

Camazine, S., et al. (2001). Self-Organization in Biological Systems. Princeton University Press.

Campbell, D. T. (1974). Downward causation in hierarchically organized biological systems. In F. J. Ayala & T. Dobzhansky (eds.), Studies in the Philosophy of Biology. University of California Press.

Chadwick, K. H., & Leenhouts, H. P. (1973). A molecular theory of cell survival. Physics in Medicine & Biology, 18(1), 78–87.

Chernet, B. T., & Levin, M. (2013). Transmembrane voltage potential is an essential cellular parameter for the detection & control of tumor development in a Xenopus model. Disease Models & Mechanisms, 6(3), 595–607.

Chis, O. T., Banga, J. R., & Balsa-Canto, E. (2011). Structural identifiability of systems biology models. PLoS ONE, 6(11), e27755.

Cole, K. S., & Cole, R. H. (1941). Dispersion & absorption in dielectrics. Journal of Chemical Physics, 9(4), 341–351.

Coutard, H. (1932). Roentgen therapy of epitheliomas of the tonsillar region, hypopharynx, & larynx from 1920 to 1926. American Journal of Roentgenology, 28, 313–331.

Curtis, S. B. (1986). Lethal and potentially lethal lesions induced by radiation — a unified repair model. *Radiation Research*, 106(2), 252–270.

Davies, P. C. W. (2012). The epigenome & top-down causation. Interface Focus, 2(1), 42–48.

Davies, P. C. W. (2019). The Demon in the Machine. University of Chicago Press.

Davies, P. C. W., & Lineweaver, C. H. (2011). Cancer tumors as Metazoa 1.0: tapping genes of ancient ancestors. Physical Biology, 8(1), 015001.

Demaria, S., & Formenti, S. C. (2015). Radiation as an immunological adjuvant: current evidence on dose & fractionation. Frontiers in Oncology, 5, 153.

Dewey, D. L., & Boag, J. W. (1959). Modification of the oxygen effect when bacteria are given large pulses of radiation. Nature, 183(4673), 1450–1451.

Doan, N., Theroux, A., Ramdas, T., & Gershman, S. J. (2026). Associative learning in the protozoan Stentor coeruleus. bioRxiv, 2026-02.

Durant, F., et al. (2017). Long-term, stochastic editing of regenerative anatomy via targeting endogenous bioelectric gradients. Biophysical Journal, 112(10), 2231–2243.

Ellis, G. F. R. (2012). Top-down causation & emergence: some comments on mechanisms. Interface Focus, 2(1), 126–140.

Favaudon, V., et al. (2014). Ultrahigh dose-rate FLASH irradiation increases the differential response between normal & tumor tissue in mice. Science Translational Medicine, 6(245), 245ra93.

Fernando, C. T., et al. (2009). Molecular circuits for associative learning in single-celled organisms. Journal of The Royal Society Interface, 6(38), 463–469.

Ferrell, J. E. (2002). Self-perpetuating states in signal transduction: positive feedback, double-negative feedback & bistability. Current Opinion in Cell Biology, 14(2), 140–148.

Flavahan, W. A., Gaskell, E., & Bernstein, B. E. (2017). Epigenetic plasticity & the hallmarks of cancer. Science, 357(6348), eaal2380.

Fowler, J. F. (1989). The linear-quadratic formula & progress in fractionated radiotherapy. British Journal of Radiology, 62(740), 679–694.

Fowler, J. F. (2010). 21 years of biologically effective dose. British Journal of Radiology, 83(991), 554–568.

Friedl, A. A., et al. (2022). Radiobiological mechanisms of FLASH radiotherapy. Radiotherapy & Oncology, 174, 70–76.

Friston, K. (2010). The free-energy principle: a unified brain theory? Nature Reviews Neuroscience, 11(2), 127–138.

Friston, K., FitzGerald, T., Rigoli, F., Schwartenbeck, P., & Pezzulo, G. (2017). Active inference: a process theory. Neural Computation, 29(1), 1–49.

Friston, K., Parr, T., & de Vries, B. (2017). The graphical brain: belief propagation & active inference. Network Neuroscience, 1(4), 381–414.

Garcia-Barros, M., et al. (2003). Tumor response to radiotherapy regulated by endothelial cell apoptosis. Science, 300(5622), 1155–1159.

Gatenby, R. A., & Brown, J. S. (2020). Integrating evolutionary dynamics into cancer therapy. Nature Reviews Clinical Oncology, 17(11), 675–686.

Gatenby, R. A., & Gillies, R. J. (2009). A microenvironmental model of carcinogenesis. Nature Reviews Cancer, 9(4), 239–252.

Gatenby, R. A., Silva, A. S., Gillies, R. J., & Frieden, B. R. (2009). Adaptive therapy. Cancer Research, 69(11), 4894–4903.

Goodhead, D. T. (1985). Saturable repair models of radiation action in mammalian cells. *Radiation Research*, 104(2 Suppl 8), S58–S67.

Granger, C. W. J. (1969). Investigating causal relations by econometric models & cross-spectral methods. Econometrica, 37(3), 424–438.

Grant, E. J., Ozasa, K., Preston, D. L., Suyama, A., Shimizu, Y., et al. (2012). Effects of radiation & lifestyle factors on risks of urothelial carcinoma in the Life Span Study of atomic bomb survivors. Radiation Research, 178(1), 86–98.

Grass, G. D., Krishna, N., & Kim, S. (2016). The immune mechanisms of abscopal effect in radiation therapy. Current Problems in Cancer, 40(1), 10--24.

Gray, L. H., et al. (1953). The concentration of oxygen dissolved in tissues at the time of irradiation as a factor in radiotherapy. British Journal of Radiology, 26(312), 638–648.

Greaves, M., & Maley, C. C. (2012). Clonal evolution in cancer. Nature, 481(7381), 306–313.

Griffin, R. J., et al. (2020). Spatially fractionated radiation therapy: history, present status, & future directions. Radiation Research, 194(5), 593–607.

Guerrero, M., & Li, X. A. (2004). Extending the linear-quadratic model for large fraction doses. Physics in Medicine & Biology, 49(20), 4825–4835.

Gupta, P. B., et al. (2011). Stochastic state transitions give rise to phenotypic equilibrium in populations of cancer cells. Cell, 146(4), 633--644.

Hanahan, D., & Weinberg, R. A. (2011). Hallmarks of cancer: the next generation. Cell, 144(5), 646–674.

Harper, M. (2009). The replicator equation as an inference dynamic. arXiv, 0911.1763.

Hawkins, R. B. (1994). A statistical theory of cell killing by radiation of varying linear energy transfer. *Radiation Research*, 140(3), 366–374.

Hawkins, R. B. (2003). A microdosimetric-kinetic model for the effect of non-Poisson distribution of lethal lesions on the variation of RBE with LET. *Radiation Research*, 160(1), 61–69.

Helmholtz, H. von (1867). Handbuch der Physiologischen Optik. Voss. [English translation: Treatise on Physiological Optics, 1925, Optical Society of America.

Hormuth, D. A., Chaudhuri, A., Pash, G., Lorenzo, G., Kapteyn, M., Wu, C., Lima, E. A. B. F., Yankeelov, T. E., & Willcox, K. (2023). Predictive digital twin for optimizing patient-specific radiotherapy regimens under uncertainty in high-grade gliomas. Frontiers in Artificial Intelligence, 6, 1222612.

Jacquez, J. A., & Perry, T. (1990). Parameter estimation: local identifiability of parameters. American Journal of Physiology, 258(4), E727--E736.

Jain, R. K. (1987). Transport of molecules in the tumor interstitium. Cancer Research, 47(12), 3039–3051.

Jaynes, E. T. (1957). Information theory & statistical mechanics. Physical Review, 106(4), 620–630.

Jeffreys, H. (1961). Theory of Probability (3rd ed.). Oxford University Press.

Jeggo, P. A., & Löbrich, M. (2007). DNA double-strand break repair & its role in genomic instability & cancer. Oncogene, 26(56), 7717–7719.

Joiner, M. C., & van der Kogel, A. J. (2018). Basic Clinical Radiobiology (5th ed.). CRC Press.

Jordan, M. I., et al. (1999). An introduction to variational methods for graphical models. Machine Learning, 37(2), 183–233.

Junttila, M. R., & de Sauvage, F. J. (2013). Influence of tumor microenvironment heterogeneity on therapeutic response. Nature, 501(7467), 346–354.

Kaelbling, L. P., Littman, M. L., & Cassandra, A. R. (1998). Planning & acting in partially observable stochastic domains. Artificial Intelligence, 101(1–2), 99–134.

Kalman, R. E. (1960). A new approach to linear filtering & prediction problems. Journal of Basic Engineering, 82(1), 35–45.

Kass, R. E., & Raftery, A. E. (1995). Bayes factors. Journal of the American Statistical Association, 90(430), 773--795.

Kellerer, A. M., & Rossi, H. H. (1972). The theory of dual radiation action. Current Topics in Radiation Research Quarterly, 8, 85–158.

Kirkpatrick, J. P., Meyer, J. J., & Marks, L. B. (2008). The linear-quadratic model is inappropriate for high doses per fraction. Seminars in Radiation Oncology, 18(4), 240–243.

Kitano, H. (2002). Systems biology: a brief overview. Science, 295(5560), 1662–1664.

Koopmans, T. C. (1949). Identification problems in economic model construction. Econometrica, 17(2), 125–144.

Kutcher, G. J., & Burman, C. (1989). Calculation of complication probability factors for non-uniform normal tissue irradiation. International Journal of Radiation Oncology Biology Physics, 16(6), 1623–1630.

Labarbe, R., et al. (2020). Modeling radiolytic oxygen depletion in FLASH radiotherapy. Radiotherapy & Oncology, 150, 136–142.

Le Bihan, D., et al. (1988). Separation of diffusion & perfusion in intravoxel incoherent motion MR imaging. Radiology, 168(2), 497–505.

Levin, M. (2014). Molecular bioelectricity: how endogenous voltage potentials control cell behavior & instruct pattern regulation in vivo. Molecular Biology of the Cell, 25(24), 3835–3850.

Levin, M. (2021). Bioelectric signaling: reprogrammable circuits underlying embryogenesis, regeneration, & cancer. Cell, 184(8), 1971–1989.

Levin, M., et al. (2021). Endogenous bioelectric signaling networks: exploiting voltage gradients for control of growth & form. Annual Review of Biomedical Engineering, 23, 295–322.

Lobikin, M., et al. (2012). Early, noncell-autonomous cell death broadens the capacity for pattern regulation during planarian regeneration. FASEB Journal, 26(11), 4445–4457.

Lucas, R. E. (1976). Econometric policy evaluation: a critique. Carnegie-Rochester Conference Series on Public Policy, 1, 19--46.

Ludwig, D., Jones, D. D., & Holling, C. S. (1978). Qualitative analysis of insect outbreak systems: the spruce budworm & forest. Journal of Animal Ecology, 47(1), 315--332.

Lyman, J. T. (1985). Complication probability as assessed from dose-volume histograms. Radiation Research, 8(Suppl), S13–19.

MacKay, D. J. C. (2003). Information Theory, Inference, & Learning Algorithms. Cambridge University Press.

Marshall, S. M., et al. (2021). Identifying molecules as biosignatures with assembly theory & mass spectrometry. Nature Communications, 12, 3033

Marusyk, A., Almendro, V., & Polyak, K. (2012). Intra-tumour heterogeneity: a looking glass for cancer? Nature Reviews Cancer, 12(5), 323–334.

Marusyk, A., et al. (2014). Non-cell-autonomous driving of tumour growth supports sub-clonal heterogeneity. Nature, 514(7520), 54--58.

Mohiuddin, M., et al. (1999). Spatially fractionated radiation therapy in the treatment of large tumors. International Journal of Radiation Oncology Biology Physics, 45(3), 721–727.

Montay-Gruel, P., et al. (2017). Long-term neurocognitive benefits of FLASH radiotherapy. Proceedings of the National Academy of Sciences, 114(27), 7257–7262.

Mukherjee, S. (2010). The Emperor of All Maladies: A Biography of Cancer. Scribner.

Mukherjee, S. (2016). The Gene: An Intimate History. Scribner.

Mukherjee, S. (2022). The Song of the Cell: An Exploration of Medicine & the New Human. Scribner.

Nowak, M. A. (2006). Evolutionary Dynamics: Exploring the Equations of Life. Harvard University Press.

Orton, C. G. (2022). A brief history of fractionation in external-beam radiotherapy. Medical Physics International, Special Issue: History of Medical Physics, 8, 1001–1010.

Osswald, M., et al. (2015). Brain tumour cells interconnect to a functional & resistant network. Nature, 528(7580), 93–8.

Oviedo, N. J., et al. (2010). Long-range neural & gap junction protein-mediated cues control polarity during planarian regeneration. Developmental Biology, 339(1), 188–199.

Park, C., et al. (2008). Universal survival curve & single fraction equivalent dose. International Journal of Radiation Oncology Biology Physics, 70(3), 847–852.

Parr, T., & Friston, K. J. (2019). Generalised free energy & active inference. Biological Cybernetics, 113(5–6), 495–513.

Pezzulo, G., & Levin, M. (2016). Top-down models in biology: explanation & control of complex living systems above the molecular level. Journal of the Royal Society Interface, 13(124), 20160555.

Pigozzi, F., Cirrito, T., & Levin, M. (2025). AI-Guided Resetting of Memories in Gene Regulatory Network Models: biomedical & evolutionary implications. bioRxiv, 2025-09.

Pigozzi, F., Goldstein, A., & Levin, M. (2025). Associative conditioning in gene regulatory network models increases integrative causal emergence. Communications Biology, 8(1), 1027.

Pineau, J., Gordon, G., & Thrun, S. (2003). Point-based value iteration: an anytime algorithm for POMDPs. International Joint Conference on Artificial Intelligence, 1025–1032.

Potters, L., et al. (2004). Stereotactic body radiation therapy: a proposed definition. International Journal of Radiation Oncology Biology Physics, 58(5), 1662–1667.

Pratx, G., & Kapp, D. S. (2019). A computational model of radiolytic oxygen depletion during FLASH irradiation. Radiotherapy & Oncology, 138, 48–55.

Prise, K. M., & O'Sullivan, J. M. (2009). Radiation-induced bystander signalling in cancer therapy. Nature Reviews Cancer, 9(5), 351–360.

Radiation Effects Research Foundation (RERF). (2007). Life Span Study of atomic bomb survivors: Report 14. Radiation Research, 167(4), 381–393.

Raue, A., et al. (2009). Structural & practical identifiability analysis of partially observed dynamical models. Bioinformatics, 25(15), 1923–1929.

Regaud, C. (1922). Influence de la durée d'irradiation sur les effets déterminés dans le testicule par le Radium. Comptes Rendus de la Société de Biologie, 86, 787–790.

Reynders, K., et al. (2019). The abscopal effect of radiation therapy: a systematic review. Radiation Oncology, 14(1), 1--11.

Safron, A. (2020). An integrated world modeling theory (IWMT) of consciousness. Frontiers in Artificial Intelligence, 3, 30.

Safron, A. (2021). The radically embodied conscious cybernetic bayesian brain. Entropy, 23(6), 783.

Salvioli, M., Garjani, H., Satouri, M., Broom, M, et al. (2024). Stackelberg evolutionary games of cancer treatment: what treatment strategy to choose if cancer can be stabilised? Dynamic Games & Applications. https://doi.org/10.1007/s13235-024-00609-z

Sargent, T. J. (1976). The observational equivalence of natural & unnatural rate theories of macroeconomics. Journal of Political Economy, 84(3), 631–640.

Scholz, M., & Kraft, G. (1996). Track structure and the calculation of biological effects of heavy charged particles. *Advances in Space Research*, 18(1–2), 5–14.

Schreiber, T. (2000). Measuring information transfer. Physical Review Letters, 85(2), 461–464.

Shaffer, S. M., et al. (2017). Rare cell variability & drug-induced reprogramming as a mode of cancer drug resistance. Nature, 546(7658), 431–435.

Shannon, C. E. (1948). A mathematical theory of communication. Bell System Technical Journal, 27(3), 379–423.

Sharma, A., et al. (2023). Assembly theory explains & quantifies selection & evolution. Nature, 622(7982), 321–328.

Sharma, S. V., et al. (2010). A chromatin-mediated reversible drug-tolerant state in cancer cell subpopulations. Cell, 141(1), 69–80.

Silver, D., et al. (2016). Mastering the game of Go with deep neural networks & tree search. Nature, 529(7587), 484–489.

Stein, A., Salvioli, M., Garjani, H., Dubbeldam, J., Viossat, Y., Brown, J. S., & Staňková, K. (2023). Stackelberg evolutionary game theory: how to manage evolving systems. Philosophical Transactions of the Royal Society B, 378(1876), 20210495.

Thames, H. D. (1988). Early fractionation methods & the origins of the NSD concept. Acta Oncologica, 27(2), 89–103.

Thrun, S., Burgard, W., & Fox, D. (2005). Probabilistic Robotics. MIT Press.

Timmerman, R. D., et al. (2010). Stereotactic body radiation therapy for inoperable early stage lung cancer. JAMA, 303(11), 1070–1076.

Tobias, C. A. (1985). The repair-misrepair model in radiobiology: comparison to other models. *Radiation Research*, 104(2 Suppl 8), S77–S95.

Tononi, G. (2004). An information integration theory of consciousness. BMC Neuroscience, 5(1), 42.

Tononi, G., Boly, M., Massimini, M., & Koch, C. (2016). Integrated information theory: from consciousness to its physical substrate. Nature Reviews Neuroscience, 17(7), 450–461.

Tuszynski, J., et al. (2022). Bioelectric dysregulation in cancer initiation, promotion, & progression. Frontiers in Oncology, 12, 846917.

Tyson, J. J., & Novak, B. (2010). Functional motifs in biochemical reaction networks. Annual Review of Physical Chemistry, 61, 219–240.

Vaitheeswaran, R. (2026a). A predictive framework for detecting non-independent tumor dynamics in longitudinal MR-guided radiotherapy. Preprints. doi:10.20944/preprints202603.2255.v1

Vaitheeswaran, R. (2026b). FLASH radiotherapy as a state transition: a memory-modulated oxygen depletion model. Preprints. doi:10.20944/preprints202603.2392.v2

Vaitheeswaran, R. (2026c). On the Observability and Structural Identifiability of Radiobiological Models and the Case for Latent-State Adaptive Control. Preprints. doi: 10.20944/preprints202605.0822.v1

Villaverde, A. F., & Banga, J. R. (2016). Structural identifiability of dynamic systems biology models. PLoS Computational Biology, 12(6), e1005153.

Vincent, M. (2012). Cancer: a de-repression of a default survival program common to all cells. BioEssays, 34(1), 72–82.

Vozenin, M. C., et al. (2019). The advantage of FLASH radiotherapy confirmed in mini-pig & cat-cancer patients. Clinical Cancer Research, 25(1), 35–42.

Webb, S. (1994). Optimum parameters in a model for tumour control probability including interpatient heterogeneity. Physics in Medicine & Biology, 39(11), 1895–1914.

Withers, H. R. (1975). The four R's of radiotherapy. In J. T. Lett & H. Adler (Eds.), Advances in Radiation Biology (Vol. 5, pp. 241–271). Academic Press.

Zhang, H., et al. (2020). Spatially fractionated radiation therapy: history, present & future. Clinical & Translational Radiation Oncology, 20, 1–10.

Zhang, J., et al. (2017). Integrating evolutionary dynamics into treatment of metastatic castrate-resistant prostate cancer. Nature Communications, 8(1), 1816.

www.ingramcontent.com/pod-product-compliance
Lightning Source LLC
LaVergne TN
LVHW090307210926
848480LV00001B/161